CONTENTS

ANITA BEAN'S
SPORTS NUTRITION
FOR YOUNG ATHLETES

A & C Black • London

Note

Whilst every effort has been made to ensure that the content of this book is as technically accurate and as sound as possible, neither the author nor the publishers can accept responsibility for any injury or loss sustained as a result of the use of this material.

Published in 2010 by A & C Black Publishers Ltd
36 Soho Square, London W1D 3QY
www.acblack.com

ISBN 978 14081 2454 3

A CIP catalogue record for this book is available from the British Library.

Acknowledgements
Cover photograph © Shutterstock (back); © Getty Images (front, top); © Bananastock Ltd (front, bottom)
Inside photographs © Shutterstock 10, 12, 14, 40, 46, 51, 68, 73, 82, 84, 86, 92, 95, 98, 101, 102, 114, 122, 132, 136, 141; istock 2, 23, 43, 49, 64, 106; Punchstock 15, 18, 57, 72; Comstock 56, 107; Anita Bean v; A&C Black vii
Designed by James Watson
Commissioned by Charlotte Croft
Edited by Kate Turvey
This book is produced using paper that is made from wood grown in managed, sustainable forests. It is natural, renewable and recyclable. The logging and manufacturing processes conform to the environmental regulations of the country of origin.

Typeset in 11 on 12.5pt Adobe Garamond by Saxon Graphics Ltd, Derby

Printed and bound in Spain by GraphyCems

ACKNOWLEDGEMENTS

I would like to thank my daughters, Chloe and Lucy (pictured below), who have been the inspiration for writing this book. They are both competitive swimmers who fit a demanding daily training and eating schedule around their school and social life! I am immensely proud of their achievements. I must also thank my husband Simon, without whose support, patience and energy this book would not have been possible.

INTRODUCTION

I have been advising coaches and parents of young athletes as well as young athletes themselves (including my own children) for many years and am delighted to have this opportunity to share my knowledge and experience.

There's no doubt that what children eat affects their health as well as their performance in sport. If they eat a poor quality diet then they not only risk illness but they will not be able to train and compete to the best of their ability. But if they eat a healthy diet that provides the correct amount of energy and nutrients, then they will enjoy better health and improved performance in their sport.

The nutritional requirements of young athletes are not too dissimilar from those of non-athletes but there are a number of special considerations. The most obvious one is meeting their energy needs, which not only have to support growth and development but also their level of activity. Young athletes exercising for an hour a day may need an extra 400–500 kcal; those training for two hours or more daily may require an extra 1000 kcal. They also need proportionally more carbohydrate, more protein and more vitamins and minerals. Chapter 1, The nutritional needs of young athletes, provides practical guidance on how to plan a healthy diet for sport.

As well as ensuring they get enough fuel and are eating the right types of food, young athletes also have to consider the timing of their food and drink intake before, during and after each training session. Chapter 2, Eating for sport, explains the optimal timing of meals, snacks and drinks as well as menu suggestions.

There may also be concerns about body weight and body composition. These issues need to be treated sensitively and it is important that young athletes seek correct advice before embarking on any regime. Chapter 3, Weight and sports performance, provides sensible weight loss and weight gain strategies to help you plan their programme.

Many young athletes take supplements, such as sports drinks, vitamins and protein supplements. But often they do not know exactly what they are or how they work. In Chapter 4 I consider the evidence for the most popular supplements and tell you which ones (may) work and which ones don't.

What young athletes eat and drink in the weeks and days before a competition, as well as on the day of the competition, will make a big difference to their performance. So it's important that they have a nutrition strategy to give them the competitive edge. Chapter 5 will help you devise one.

To help you put the nutrition information into practice I have devised simple and tasty recipes for main meals, vegetarian meals, soups, desserts and baking at the end of this book. Hopefully, these will inspire you and your young athletes to get in the kitchen and get cooking!

It's not essential that young athletes eat a perfect diet all the time, but provided they get it right about 80 per cent of the time, then they will have a great chance of putting in their best performance.

I hope you find this book helpful.

Anita Bean
June 2010

01

THE NUTRITIONAL NEEDS OF YOUNG ATHLETES

How can good nutritional practices help young athletes perform better? According to the International Olympic Committee (IOC) in its 2003 Consensus statement:

The amount, composition and timing of food intake can profoundly affect sports performance. Good nutritional practice will help athletes train hard, recover quickly and adapt more effectively with less risk of illness and injury. Athletes should adopt specific nutritional strategies before and during competition to help maximise their performance.

What this means, in practice, is that a healthy diet will help young athletes:

- have more energy for training;
- increase their stamina and strength;
- recover faster;
- reduce their chances of illness and minor injuries;
- gain a competitive edge.

During childhood and adolescence, growth and development is rapid, and this places high energy and nutritional demands on the young athlete's body. Clearly, their diet needs to provide enough energy, carbohydrate, fat, protein, vitamins and minerals to fuel growth as well as training and recovery. The energy and nutrient requirements for boys and girls aged 4–18 years are shown in Tables 1.1 and 1.2. These values should cover the needs of 95 per cent of children. But there are no specific values for athletic children, who will almost certainly need to eat more than their non-active peers. To help you plan their food intake, this chapter provides a basic guide to young athletes' nutritional needs.

Table 1.1 Dietary reference values for boys aged 4–18

	Dietary reference value (DRV)	4–6 years	7–10 years	11–14 years	15–18 years
Energy	Estimated average requirement (EAR)	1715 kcal	1979 kcal	2220 kcal	2755 kcal
Fat	Max. 35% energy	67 g	77 g	86 g	107 g
Saturated fat	Max. 11% energy	21 g	24 g	27 g	34 g
Carbohydrate	Min. 50% energy	229 g	263 g	296 g	367 g
Added sugars*	Max. 11% energy	50 g	58 g	65 g	81 g
Fibre**	8 g per 1000 kcal	14 g	16 g	18 g	22 g
Protein		19.7 g	28 g	42 g	55 g
Iron		6.1 mg	8.7 mg	11.3 mg	11.3 mg
Zinc		6.5 mg	7.0 mg	9.0 mg	9.5 mg
Calcium		450 mg	550 mg	1000 mg	1000 mg
Vitamin A		500 mcg	500 mcg	600 mcg	700 mcg
Vitamin C		30 mg	30 mg	35 mg	40 mg
Folate		100 mcg	150 mcg	200 mcg	200 mcg
Salt***		3 g	5 g	6 g	6 g

Source: Department of Health (1991)

Notes
* Non-milk extrinsic sugars
** Proportion of adult DRV (18 g), i.e. 8 g/1000 kcal
*** Scientific Advisory Committee on Nutrition (2003)

Table 1.2 Dietary reference values for girls aged 4–18

	Dietary reference value (DRV)	4–6 years	7–10 years	11–14 years	15–18 years
Energy	Estimated average requirement (EAR)	1545 kcal	1740 kcal	1845 kcal	2110 kcal
Fat	Max. 35% energy	60 g	68 g	72 g	82 g
Saturated fat	Max. 11% energy	19 g	21 g	23 g	26 g
Carbohydrate	Min. 50% energy	206 g	232 g	246 g	281 g
Added sugars*	Max. 11% energy	45 g	51 g	54 g	62 g
Fibre**	8 g per 1000 kcal	12 g	14 g	15 g	17 g
Protein		19.7 g	28 g	41 g	45 g
Iron		6.1 mg	8.7 mg	14.8 mg	14.8 mg
Zinc		6.5 mg	7.0 mg	9.0 mg	7.0 mg
Calcium		450 mg	550 mg	800 mg	800 mg
Vitamin A		500 mcg	500 mcg	600 mcg	600 mcg
Vitamin C		30 mg	30 mg	35 mg	40 mg
Folate		100 mcg	150 mcg	200 mcg	200 mcg
Salt***		3 g	5 g	6 g	6 g

Source: Department of Health (1991)

Notes
* Non-milk extrinsic sugars
** Proportion of adult DRV (18 g), i.e. 8 g/1000 kcal
*** Scientific Advisory Committee on Nutrition (2003)

ENERGY, CALORIES – WHAT'S THE DIFFERENCE?

Most people think of energy as good, calories bad. In fact, they refer to the same thing! Calories are a measure of energy, whether it's the energy content of food or the energy cost of exercise. When we talk about calories in the everyday sense, we actually mean kilocalories (1000 calories = 1 kilocalorie or 1 kcal). This is what you'll see on the nutrition information panel on food labels and physical activity charts.

WHAT IS THE PHYSICAL ACTIVITY LEVEL (PAL)?

The PAL is the total energy cost of a person's physical activity throughout the day, expressed as a ratio of their basal metabolic rate (BMR). The more active they are, the higher the PAL. Most young athletes would probably have a PAL of 2.0. Table 1.3 describes a range of PALs.

Table 1.3 Physical activity level (PAL)

Physical activity level (PAL)	Description	Examples
1.4	Sedentary	Mainly sitting
1.5	Sedentary – moderately active	Mainly sitting/a little physical activity
1.6	Moderately active	Some walking/moderate activity
1.8	Active	Daily moderate activity
2.0	Very active	Daily intense activity or sport

How much energy do young athletes need?

The amount of energy (or calories) young athletes need to consume depends on several things: their age, their weight, how much muscle they have and how active they are. In general, the heavier they are, the more muscle they have; and the more active they are, the greater their daily expenditure, therefore the more energy they need to consume. In addition, they need an extra 60 to 100 kcal per day for growth (Department of Health, 1991).

Table 1.4 gives the estimated energy needs for 10–17 year olds for different body weights and physical activity levels (PALs). The BMR (*see* the box, 'What is the basal metabolic rate (BMR)?') is derived from a formula based on body weight (Schofield *et al.*, 1985).

As you can see from Table 1.4, young athletes (assuming a PAL of 2.0) have considerably higher energy needs than their non-athletic peers. For example, an athletic 65 kg boy (PAL 2.0) would need about 3612 kcal a day, while a 60 kg girl (PAL 2.0) would need 2990 kcal – almost an extra 900 kcal compared with non-athletic teenagers with the same body weight (PAL 1.4–1.5).

Unfortunately, there are no published data on the energy cost of various activities for children, but it is possible to make an estimate by extrapolating from adult values. Table 1.5 provides values for adults with different body weights, and should give you a rough idea of how much energy young athletes burn during training. Bear in mind, though, that these values may underestimate the actual energy burn for younger children. Younger children use more energy per kg body weight than do teenagers and adults (Macdougall *et al.*, 1982). Generally, the younger the child the higher the relative energy cost. A 7 year old, for example, would burn 25–30 per cent more energy per kg body weight than would an adult walking or running at the same speed. This is explained by the relative 'wastefulness' of energy in children, due to lack of coordination. As their proficiency improves, though, the energy cost decreases. As a rule of thumb, for children 8–10 years old, add 20–25 per cent to the adult values; add 10–15 per cent for children aged 11–14 years.

WHAT IS THE BASAL METABOLIC RATE (BMR)?

At least 60 per cent of a person's daily energy burn is used to keep the heart beating, the organs functioning and the core body temperature stable. This is called the basal metabolic rate (BMR), and is higher for children and teenagers than for adults.

Table 1.4 Estimated average energy requirements of children and adolescents according to body weight and physical activity level

Weight (kg)	BMR kcal/d	PAL				
		1.4	1.5	1.6	1.8	2.0
Boys						
30	1189	1675	1794	1914	2153	2368
35	1278	1794	1914	2057	2297	2559
40	1366	1914	2057	2177	2464	2727
45	1455	2033	2177	2320	2632	2919
50	1543	2153	2321	2464	2775	3086
55	1632	2297	2440	2608	2943	3253
60	1720	2416	2584	2751	3086	3445
65	1809	2536	2703	2895	3254	3612
Girls						
30	1095	1531	1651	1746	1962	2201
35	1163	1627	1715	1866	2081	2321
40	1229	1722	1842	1962	2201	2464
45	1297	1818	1938	2081	2344	2584
50	1364	1913	2033	2177	2464	2727
55	1430	2009	2153	2297	2584	2871
60	1498	2105	2249	2392	2703	2990

Source: Department of Health (1991)

Table 1.5 The energy cost of various activities

Body weight (kg)	44	50	56	62	68	74
Body weight (lb)	97	110	123	137	159	163
Badminton	265	300	325	360	395	430
Basketball	365	415	460	510	565	610
Competitive	390	445	500	550	600	655
Boxing	400	455	510	565	620	675
Circuit training	350	380	410	440	470	500
Cycling @ 12 mph	360	390	425	460	495	530
Racing	450	510	570	630	690	750
Dancing	270	295	320	345	370	395
Hockey	360	405	450	500	545	590
Football	355	400	445	490	535	580
Horse riding	240	275	310	345	370	405
Rowing	600	660	720	780	830	890
Running @ 6.5 mph	425	480	535	590	650	705
@ 10 mph	620	690	765	835	900	965
Squash	515	580	645	710	785	850
Swimming: slow	230	260	290	320	350	380
Fast laps	400	445	490	535	580	625
Tennis	300	340	375	415	455	490
Weight training	350	395	440	485	530	575
Walking 5 mph	200	220	240	260	280	300

What are the best fuels for exercise?

Muscles burn a mixture of carbohydrate, fat and (to a much smaller extent) protein during exercise. The amounts and proportions of each fuel burned will depend on the intensity and duration of the activity.

As a rule of thumb, the higher the training intensity, the higher the proportion of carbohydrate used. During high-intensity aerobic activities, such as fast running or fast swimming, the muscles burn mostly carbohydrate and proportionally less fat.

During lower-intensity activities, such as jogging or slow swimming, the muscles burn fewer calories per minute and proportionally less carbohydrate.

Most of the carbohydrate is supplied by the muscles' store of glycogen. But this store is relatively small – enough to fuel perhaps 1½–2 hours of intense exercise. Once glycogen levels become depleted, exercise starts to feel much harder and fatigue sets in. Starting a training session with high levels of muscle glycogen will help delay fatigue and increase endurance.

Think of filling up a car with petrol before setting off on a journey. If you start with a full fuel tank, you will be able to travel further; if you start with low fuel levels you won't be able to travel as far. Similarly, for athletes, if they begin training with high glycogen levels they will be able to train harder and longer before reaching fatigue point. If they begin training with low glycogen levels, they will tire more easily and perform below their potential. To delay fatigue, encourage young athletes to eat a carbohydrate-rich diet during the 24–48 hours before training.

How much carbohydrate should young athletes eat each day?

This will depend on their weight – or, more accurately, the amount of muscle they are carrying – and how active they are each day. The heavier they are and the more active they are, the more carbohydrate they should eat. Table 1.6 gives the estimated carbohydrate requirements for athletes with different body weights for various activity levels. Young athletes training for up to 2 hours a day would need around 5–7 g carbohydrate for each 1 kg body weight; those training for more than 2 hours, would need 7–10 g/kg body weight/day. For example, a 60 kg athlete training for 1–2 hours each day would need 360–420 g carbohydrate daily, or 420–600 g daily if training for 2–4 hours.

Table 1.6 Carbohydrate needs for young athletes

Number of hours' exercise per day	Carbo-hydrate/kg body weight/day	Carbo-hydrate/day for a 50 kg person	Carbo-hydrate/day for a 60 kg person	Carbo-hydrate/day for a 70 kg person
0–1	5–6 g	250–300 g	300–360 g	350–420 g
1–2	6–7 g	300–350 g	360–420 g	420–490 g
3–4	7–8 g	350–400 g	420–480 g	490–560 g
4+	8–10 g	400–500 g	480–600 g	560–700 g

Tell me how to do it!

To give you an idea of how much food an athlete would need to eat, the following menu contains approximately 400 g carbohydrate – enough to fuel around 2 hours' daily exercise for someone weighing 60 kg.

Sample menu
Breakfast
2 slices of toast with margarine and honey
2 bananas

Lunch
1 large baked potato (200 g) with margarine, half a tin (200 g) of baked beans and 2 tablespoons (40 g) grated cheese
Salad
1 fruit yoghurt

Dinner
Large bowl of pasta (125 g dry weight)
Chicken breast (200g) or cheese (40g)
Vegetables

Snacks
2 pieces of fresh fruit
400 ml fruit juice
2 cereal bars
1 fruit yoghurt

Energy
2800 kcal

Carbohydrate
411 g

As a rule of thumb, young athletes should be able to meet their carbohydrate requirements by eating:

- 4–6 portions of grains/potatoes;
- 5 portions of fruit/vegetables;
- 2–4 portions of dairy products.

One portion of grains/potatoes is equivalent to two slices of bread or 150 g potatoes; a portion of fruit is equivalent to a banana, and a portion of dairy is equivalent to a glass (200 ml) of milk (*see* page 37).

Table 1.7 will help you work out how much food a young athlete should eat, as will checking the carbohydrate values on food labels.

Table 1.7 The carbohydrate content of different foods

Food	Energy (kcal)	Carbohydrate (g)
Apples (one, 100 g)	47	12
Baked beans (200 g)	162	30
Bananas (one, 100 g)	95	23
Biscuits (one, 15 g)	70	10
Bran flakes (40 g)	132	29
Bread (one slice, 35 g)	80	15
Cereal bar (one, 30 g)	140	18
Flapjacks (one, 70 g)	345	44
Jam or honey (15 g)	40	10
Milk, semi-skimmed (300 ml)	138	14
Oatcakes (one, 13 g)	54	8
Orange juice (200 ml)	72	18
Pasta (85 g dried weight)	196	64
Pitta bread (one, 60 g)	160	34
Porridge (200 g)	166	23
Potatoes (200 g)	150	34
Rice (85 g dried weight)	303	69
Roll (one, 50 g)	120	22
Shreddies (40 g)	138	31
Sweetcorn (80 g)	89	16
Weetabix (two, 40 g)	141	30
Yoghurt (one pot, 150 g)	117	21

How can I tell whether they are eating enough – or too much?

It can be tricky to judge exactly how much food young athletes should eat. In an ideal world, everyone would be guided by their appetite, and eat just the right amount of food to maintain their body weight and fuel their activities. But, in practice, it's not always easy to get it right! As a rough guide, if young athletes always seem hungry, struggle to recover fully between training sessions, and frequently lack energy while training, this suggests that they may need to step up their energy and carbohydrate intake.

Other signs that they may not be consuming enough energy and carbo-hydrate include frequent colds, infections and minor illnesses. This is because a sub-optimal intake of carbohydrate can reduce the availability of fuel to the immune cells and increase the production of stress hormones (adrenaline and cortisol), which reduces immune function. All this makes a person more susceptible to infection and illness.

On the other hand, if young athletes are putting on unwanted pounds, cutting back on carbohydrates – as well as fat – will help them lose weight. The body can store only around 400–500 g glycogen; any excess carbohydrate is converted to fat. The best way to prevent weight gain is to keep a check on portion sizes and divide their daily carbohydrate intake into several moderate-sized meals or snacks throughout the day. Make sure they don't eat all their carbohydrate in one big meal. And, if they have a tendency to gain weight easily, they should avoid snacking on 'energy dense' carbo-hydrate foods such as biscuits, crisps, sweets and chocolate.

Which are the best carbs to eat?

The best foods to eat for performance are those that contain carbohydrate along with high levels of fibre and other nutrients, such as vitamins and minerals. Encourage young athletes to opt for whole grains rather than refined versions: wholemeal bread instead of white bread; wholegrain pasta instead of ordinary pasta; wholegrain rice instead of white; and wholegrain breakfast cereals such as porridge, whole-wheat bisks (e.g. Weetabix), malted wheats (e.g. Nestlé's Shreddies), bran flakes, whole-wheat and oat flakes (e.g. Nestlé's Oats & More; Kellogg's Just Right), Nestlé's Shredded Wheat and muesli. They should also include lots of starchy vegetables, such as potatoes, sweet potatoes and sweetcorn; as well as pulses (beans and lentils), which provide protein as well as carbohydrate. Nutritious snack choices include fresh and dried fruit – these foods contain natural sugars as well as all-important vitamins, minerals, antioxidants and fibre.

All of these foods will provide young athletes with sustained energy. Their high fibre content means that they digest and break down more slowly than high-sugar foods (e.g. sweets, fizzy drinks) and refined starchy foods made from white flour (e.g. white bread). This means that they are digested more slowly and release glucose into the bloodstream over a longer period. Eating them with protein, such as fish, cheese or milk, would produce an even more gradual energy release. So, eating breakfast cereal with milk, potato with tuna, or bread with cheese, will fuel the body for longer.

CARBOHYDRATE-RICH FOODS AT A GLANCE

Good main meal choices	Good snack choices	Choose less often
Wholegrain pasta Wholegrain rice Baked or boiled potatoes Sweet potatoes Sweetcorn Wholegrain bread, rolls, pitta, wraps Wholegrain breakfast cereals Porridge/oatmeal Beans, chickpeas, lentils	Fresh fruit, e.g. apples, pears, oranges, peaches, apricots, bananas, grapes, kiwi fruit, strawberries, mango Dried fruit, e.g. raisins, apricots, figs Rice cakes Oat cakes Wholegrain crackers Cereal bars Crumpets Plain popcorn	White bread and rolls, French bread and bagels White rice High-sugar breakfast cereals

Is sugar good or bad for young athletes?

Sugar is a carbohydrate, which means it is an energy source for the body. Like starch, it can be used to fuel exercise, convert into glycogen or turn into fat. It is absorbed rapidly into the bloodstream, which can be useful during long, intense training sessions when the muscles may run low on glycogen and need extra fuel quickly. Consuming sugar (for example, a sports drink, a cereal bar or dried fruit) would be beneficial for performance when exercising hard for longer than an hour, but unnecessary for shorter sessions (*see* Chapter 2, page 45). Sugar-containing drinks and foods may also be beneficial for refuelling muscles during the two-hour period after exercise (*see* Chapter 2, page 54).

However, there are many myths when it comes to sugar and performance. For example, many people believe that consuming high-sugar foods or drinks will give them extra energy for exercise. I frequently see young athletes munching sweets and chocolate bars on their way to training sessions, or swigging sugary drinks just before setting out. In fact, researchers have shown that the opposite holds true – consuming sugar before exercise, does *not* improve performance or stamina (Burke *et al.*, 1998; Wu and Williams, 2006). The problem is that eating lots of sugar triggers high levels of insulin in the bloodstream, which transports sugar out of the bloodstream rapidly, leaving the athlete with less available energy. This rebound effect can make athletes feel tired, weak and light-headed. Instead, encourage them to eat a healthy meal based on potatoes, wholegrain bread or pasta two to four hours before training, or a snack based on fruit or cereals 30 minutes before exercise (*see* Chapter 2, page 43–44).

Remember that sugar is harmful for teeth and lacks other useful nutrients, so young athletes should keep it to a minimum in their day-to-day diet, particularly between meals when they can do the most damage to the teeth. If they must have a sweet treat, it is better that they consume sugar at mealtimes when it is less likely to cause decay. Sugary drinks and sports drinks are highly acidic and can, over time, cause a thinning of the enamel and a change in the texture, shape and appearance of teeth. Minimise the risk of acid erosion by getting young athletes to use a drinks bottle with a spout, direct the drink towards the back of the mouth and, ideally, have some water afterwards to wash away the acid and sugar.

Sugar that occurs naturally in foods such as fruit, vegetables and milk is locked in to the structure of the food and tends to be less harmful to the teeth. These foods supply lots of other nutrients, so are a healthier choice.

How much sugar should young athletes eat?

There are no official dietary guidelines (although this is currently under review at the time of going to print) but the guideline daily amount (GDA) for 'added' (or 'non-milk extrinsic sugars', NME) sugars is 11 per cent of the daily energy intake. However, food labels do not distinguish between 'added' and 'natural' sugars (such as those found in fruit and milk), and give you the 'total sugar' sugar content of the product. The GDA for total sugar is 20 per cent of daily energy. Table 1.8 shows the GDA for different ages. These values apply to non-athletic children. As athletic children have higher energy needs they can consume a little more sugar, although this should still be within 20 per cent of daily energy intake.

Table 1.8 Guideline daily amounts for sugar

	11–14 years	15–18 years
Girls		
Total sugars	90 g	105 g
NME sugars	50 g	60 g
Boys		
Total sugars	110 g	140 g
NME sugars	60 g	75 g

Check food labels for sugar. The Food Standard Agency's 'traffic light' labelling scheme says that foods containing more than 15 g sugar per 100 g, or drinks containing more than 7.5 g sugar per 100 ml, are 'high in sugar' (and would have a red label), and should be kept to a minimum.

SUGAR GUIDE FOR ATHLETES

- Young athletes should save their sugar for exercise. During training sessions lasting more than an hour, squash, diluted fruit juice and sports drinks, dried fruit and cereal bars will help fuel tiring muscles and improve endurance.
- At other times, if they want something sweet, they should opt for foods that contain additional nutrients: fresh fruit, dried fruit, fruit yoghurt, fruit juice, smoothies, cereal bars and breakfast cereal.
- Set a sensible daily limit of two or three portions for high-sugar foods – e.g. sweets, chocolate, biscuits, cakes and puddings (*see* pages 35–36).
- They should drink water after eating or drinking anything sugary, to help wash the sugar away, or chew gum to stimulate the production of saliva, which can neutralise the acid.

How much protein do young athletes need?

Their diet needs to cover their protein requirements for growth and development, for day-to-day repair and maintenance of body proteins, as well as a little extra for fuelling intense exercise. Non-athletic children aged 13–18 years need around 0.85–1 g protein for each 1 kg of body weight, or about 55 g for someone weighing 60 kg (Department of Health, 1991). There are no published values for young athletes – only for adult athletes – but it is estimated that they need more than non-athletes, around 1.2 to 1.4 g per 1 kg body weight – that's 72–84 g for someone weighing 60 kg (Boisseau *et al.*, 2007). Adult athletes require a similar amount, between 1.2 and 1.7 g protein/kg body weight (IAAF, 2007). This goes to repair the muscle proteins broken down during intense exercise, and also to make new muscle tissue.

The protein needs for young athletes of different body weights are given in Table 1.9.

Table 1.9 Protein needs of young athletes

Body weight	Daily protein requirement
44 kg (97 lb)	53–62 g
50 kg (110 lb)	60–70 g
56 kg (123 lb)	67–78 g
62 kg (137 kg)	74–87 g
68 kg (159 lb)	82–95 g

What are the best ways to get protein?

Protein is found in many foods. The richest sources include lean meat such as chicken and turkey, fish, eggs, cheese, milk, yoghurt, beans, lentils, nuts, soya and Quorn (a mycoprotein). Other useful sources include cereal-based foods, such as bread, pasta

and breakfast cereals. Including two to three portions of protein-rich foods daily makes it relatively easy for young athletes to meet their daily requirement. You can work out the protein content of a young athlete's diet by checking Table 1.10, as well as the nutrition information on food labels.

What are 'good' and 'bad' fats?

'Good' fats are the unsaturated fats – the monounsaturates and polyunsaturates, found in nuts, seeds, olives (and their oils) and fish.

'Bad' fats are saturated fats and trans fats, which have been linked to increased risk of heart disease and cancer.

Table 1.11 Good and bad fats

Good fats	Bad fats
Monounsaturated fats: olive oil, rapeseed oil, avocados, nuts, peanut butter	*Saturated fats:* fatty meats, burgers, sausages, butter, palm oil, biscuits, cakes, cheese
Polyunsaturated fats: sunflower oil, corn oil, sunflower margarine, nuts, seeds	*Trans fats:* some margarines and spreads, biscuits, pastries, pies, cakes, takeaway fried food
Omega-3 fats: sardines, salmon, mackerel, pilchards, walnuts, pumpkin seeds, omega-3 eggs	

Good fats

Monounsaturated fats help lower 'bad' LDL (low-density lipoprotein) cholesterol levels while maintaining levels of 'good' HDL (high-density lipoprotein), which helps cut heart disease and cancer risk. They are found in olive oil, rapeseed and soya oil, avocados, nuts, peanut butter and seeds.

Polyunsaturated fats include omega-3 and omega-6 fats.

Omega-3 fatty acids include alpha linolenic acid (ALA, found in walnuts, pumpkin seeds, flaxseeds and rapeseed oil), eicosapentanoic acid (EPA) and docosahexanoic acid (DHA), the latter two are both found only in oily fish (sardines, mackerel, salmon, fresh tuna, trout, herring). In the body, ALA can be converted into EPA and DHA, which are needed for the proper functioning of the brain, protect against heart disease and stroke, and may help prevent memory loss and treat depression. For athletes, they help increase the delivery of oxygen to muscles, improve endurance, speed recovery, and reduce inflammation and joint stiffness. The minimum requirement is 0.9 g per day, which can come from one portion (140 g) of oily fish a week or one tablespoon of omega-3-rich oil daily.

Omega-6 fatty acids include linolenic acid and gamma linolenic acid (GLA) found in sunflower, safflower, corn, groundnut and olive oils, and margarine-type spreads made with them, peanuts and peanut butter, and sunflower and sesame seeds. Most children get plenty of omega-6s but not enough omega-3s.

Bad fats

Saturated fats are found in animal fats as well as products made with palm oil. They have no beneficial role in the body (apart from being a source of energy). They raise blood cholesterol levels and increase the risk of heart disease. However, it would be impractical to cut them out altogether, so young athletes should try to stick to an intake less than the GDA: 30 g for males and 20 g for females.

Main sources include fatty meats, full-fat dairy products, butter, lard, palm oil and palm kernel oil (both labelled as 'vegetable fat' on foods), and biscuits, cakes and desserts made with palm or palm kernel oil or 'vegetable fat'.

Trans fats are formed artificially during the commercial process of hydrogenation, which converts unsaturated oils into solid spreads (hydrogenated fats or oils) for making biscuits, desserts and pastry. Trans fats increase LDL ('bad') cholesterol levels and lower HDL ('good') cholesterol, and harden and stiffen the arteries, which increases the risk of heart disease.

Young athletes should try to avoid these fats completely by checking for hydrogenated oils and partially hydrogenated oils on the ingredients list on food packages.

What do vitamins and minerals do?

Vitamins and minerals are substances that are needed in tiny amounts to enable the body to work properly and prevent illness. There are 13 different vitamins, which are involved in numerous processes, including energy production, nerve and muscle function, the immune system, brain function, and healthy growth and development. Some vitamins – the B vitamins and vitamin C – must be provided by the diet each day, as they cannot be stored. The 15 minerals have mainly structural roles, such as bone strength, and regulatory roles, such as fluid balance and muscle contraction. Table 1.12 gives more details of the functions, requirements, sources and side-effects of vitamins and minerals.

WHAT ARE RDAs?

You'll see recommended daily amounts (RDAs) on food and supplement labels, which are estimates of nutrient requirements set by the EU and designed to cover the needs of the majority (97 per cent) of the general population. The amounts are designed to prevent deficiency symptoms, but also allow for storage and individual variation, as well as covering differences in needs from one person to the next. They do not necessarily cover the needs of people who are physically very active, so regard them as a rough guide only.

Do athletes need extra vitamins and minerals?

Athletes' requirements for most vitamins and minerals are higher than those of non-active people. Many of them are involved in producing energy and helping the body recover after exercise. Some are involved in repairing cells broken down during exercise, making new muscle tissue, making red blood cells and protecting cells against the harmful free radicals produced during exercise.

The best way for young athletes to get their vitamins and minerals is by eating a nutrient-rich diet, rather than taking supplements. Make sure they include lots of fruit and vegetables – at least five daily portions – and wholegrain cereals (rather than white versions), and keep low-nutrient foods such as sugary snacks, fried foods, fast foods and soft drinks to a minimum.

Can vitamin and mineral supplements improve their performance?

It is tempting to believe that supplements will benefit an athlete's performance but, in fact, there's little scientific evidence to support their use (IOC, 2004; Lukaski, 2004). According to a 2009 review of evidence, supplements are not needed if athletes are eating a varied diet that matches their energy needs (Rodriquez *et al.*, 2009). Only if their diet is unbalanced (e.g. lacking fresh fruit and vegetables; or any major food group), should you consider supplements. In general, young athletes should aim to get their vitamins and minerals from their diet rather than from supplements. Nutrients are absorbed better from food, where there are also other important components such as fibre, protein and essential fats. Supplements are not a substitute for an unhealthy diet.

Table 1.12 A guide to vitamins and minerals

Vitamin/ mineral	How much?*	Why is it needed?	What happens if we get too little?	What are the best food sources?	Side-effects of excessive intake?
Vitamin A	700 mcg (boys) 600 mcg (girls) FSA recommends 1500 mcg max.	Needed for growth and development in children; helps vision in dim light; keeps the skin, hair and eyes healthy; keeps the linings of organs such as the lungs and digestive tract healthy; helps the body to fight infections	Poor vision, dry skin, impaired growth in children, and an increased susceptibility to infection	Liver, cheese, oily fish, eggs, butter, margarine	Liver and bone damage; can harm unborn children in pregnant women (avoid during pregnancy)
Beta-carotene	No official RNI SUL = 7 mg	Converts into vitamin A, a powerful antioxidant that may protect against certain cancers and heart disease		Dark-green vegetables such as spinach and watercress, and yellow, orange and red fruits such as carrots, tomatoes, dried apricots, sweet potatoes and mangoes	Excessive doses of beta-carotene can cause harmless orange tinge to skin; reversible

Vitamin/ mineral	How much?*	Why is it needed?	What happens if we get too little?	What are the best food sources?	Side-effects of excessive intake?
Thiamin	0.9 mg (11–14 y/o boys) 1.1 mg (15–18 y/o boys) 0.7 mg (11–14 y/o girls) 0.8 mg (15–18 y/o girls) no SUL; FSA recommends 100 mg	Converts carbohydrates to energy; keeps nervous system and the heart healthy	Tiredness, poor appetite, headaches, muscle fatigue, poor concentration, depression, irritability and heart problems	Wholemeal bread, fortified breakfast cereals, nuts, pulses, meat	Excess is excreted, so toxicity is rare
Riboflavin	0.9 mg (11–14 y/o boys) 1.1 mg (15–18 y/o boys) 0.7 mg (11–14 y/o girls) 0.8 mg (15–18 y/o girls) no SUL; FSA recommends 40 mg	Converts carbohydrates, fats and protein into energy	Poor wound healing, and skin, eye and mouth problems such as watery, bloodshot eyes, flaky and dry skin, chapped lips and a sore tongue	Milk and dairy products, meat, eggs	Excess is excreted (producing yellow urine!), so toxicity is rare

Vitamin/ mineral	How much?*	Why is it needed?	What happens if we get too little?	What are the best food sources?	Side-effects of excessive intake?
Niacin	15 mg (11–14 y/o boys) 18 mg (15–18 y/o boys) 12 mg (11–14 y/o girls) 14 mg (15–18 y/o girls) SUL = 17 mg	Converts carbohydrates, fats and protein into energy	Skin problems, weakness, fatigue and loss of appetite	Meat and offal, nuts, milk and dairy products, eggs, wholegrain cereals	Excess is excreted; high doses may cause hot flushes
Folate	200 mcg for 11–18 y/o boys and girls	Formation of red blood cells; works with vitamin B12 for growth and the reproduction of cells	Tiredness, apathy and depression	Dark-green leafy vegetables, oranges, fortified breakfast cereals and bread, yeast extract, nuts and pulses	May mask symptoms of a B12 deficiency

Vitamin/ mineral	How much?*	Why is it needed?	What happens if we get too little?	What are the best food sources?	Side-effects of excessive intake?
Vitamin C	35 mg for 11–14 y/o boys and girls 40 mg for 15–18 y/o boys and girls SUL = 1000 mg	Formation of collagen, which constitutes connective tissue; needed for healthy bones, teeth, blood vessels, gums and teeth; promotes immune function; helps iron absorption	Loss of appetite, muscle cramps, dry skin, bleeding gums, bruising, nose bleeds, infections and poor wound healing; in severe cases scurvy develops	Fruit and vegetables (e.g. raspberries, blackcurrants, kiwi fruit, oranges, peppers, broccoli, cabbage, tomatoes)	Excess is excreted; doses over 2 g may lead to diarrhoea and excess urine formation; high doses (> 2 g) may cause vitamin C to behave as a pro-oxidant (enhance free radical damage)
Vitamin D	No RNI SUL = 25 mcg	Needed for strong bones (with calcium and phosphorus), helps to absorb calcium, and may help to prevent osteoporosis in later life	Reduced absorption of calcium (increasing the risk of osteoporosis); deficiency in babies and toddlers leads to soft bones and the development of rickets	Sunlight, oily fish, eggs, liver, fortified breakfast cereals and margarine	Toxicity rare; very high doses may cause high blood pressure, irregular heart beat; excessive thirst

Vitamin/ mineral	How much?*	Why is it needed?	What happens if we get too little?	What are the best food sources?	Side-effects of excessive intake?
Vitamin E	No RNI in UK 10 mg in EU SUL = 540 mg	Antioxidant that helps protect against heart disease; promotes normal cell growth and development	Deficiency is rare	Vegetable oils, margarine, oily fish, nuts, seeds, egg yolk, avocado	Toxicity is rare
Calcium	1000 mg (11–18 y/o boys) 800 mg (11–18 y/o girls) SUL = 1500 mg	Builds bone and teeth; blood clotting; nerve and muscle function	Increased risk of osteoporosis	Milk and dairy products, sardines, dark-green leafy vegetables, pulses, nuts and seeds	High intakes may interfere with absorption of other minerals; take with magnesium and vitamin D
Iron	11.3 mg (11–18 y/o boys) 14.8 mg (11–18 y/o girls) SUL = 17 mg	Formation of red blood cells; oxygen transport; prevents anaemia	Iron deficiency; anaemia	Meat and offal, wholegrain cereals, fortified breakfast cereals, pulses, green leafy vegetables	Constipation, stomach discomfort; avoid unnecessary supplementation – may increase free radical damage

The fitness food pyramid

The components of the fitness food pyramid are described below (*see* also Table 1.13).

Fruit and vegetables
At least 5 portions a day

  Fruit and vegetables contain vitamins, minerals, fibre, antioxidants and phyto-nutrients, which are vital for health, immunity and peak performance.

Grains and potatoes
4–6+ portions a day

  The foods in this group – bread, breakfast cereals, rice, pasta, porridge oats and potatoes – provide high levels of carbohydrate. More active people will need to eat more portions or bigger portions to meet their energy needs. Aim for mostly whole-grain versions of cereals, i.e. wholegrain bread, breakfast cereals and pasta instead of 'white' versions, as these have a higher content of fibre, iron and B vitamins. The portion sizes in this group are about twice those recommended in the EatWell Plate.

Calcium-rich foods
2–4 portions a day

  The foods in this group include dairy products, nuts, pulses and tinned fish; they provide high amounts of calcium, which is needed for strong bones.

Protein-rich foods
2–4 portions a day

This group includes lean meat, chicken, turkey, fish, eggs, beans, lentils, dairy products, soya and Quorn; these provide protein as well as various different vitamins and minerals.

Healthy fats
1–2 portions a day

Omega-3 and omega-6 unsaturated fats found in nuts, seeds, rapeseed oil, olive oil, flaxseed oil, sunflower oil and oily fish are important for heart health, and for good performance and recovery after exercise.

Foods and drinks high in fats and/or sugar

These foods – biscuits, cakes, puddings, sugary drinks, chocolate and crisps – should be regarded as treats. As they provide energy but few nutrients other than fat or sugar, try to limit them to about three portions a day. They should not take the place of more nutrient-dense foods – make sure young athletes eat the recommended number of portions of the other food groups first.

Table 1.13 The fitness food pyramid

Food group	Number of portions each day	Food	Portion size
1a Vegetables	3–5	*1 portion = 80 g (about the amount you can hold in the palm of your hand)*	
		Broccoli, cauliflower	2–3 spears/florets
		Carrots	1 carrot
		Other vegetables	2 tablespoons
		Tomatoes	5 cherry tomatoes
1b Fruit	2–4	*1 portion = 80 g (about the size of a tennis ball)*	
		Apple, pear, peach, banana	1 medium fruit

Food group	Number of portions each day	Food	Portion size
		Plum, kiwi fruit, satsuma	1–2 fruits
		Strawberries	8–10
		Grapes	12–16
		Tinned fruit	3 tablespoons
		Fruit juice	1 medium glass
2 Grains and potatoes	4–6+	*1 portion = about the size of your clenched fist*	
		Bread	2 slices (60 g)
		Roll/bagel/wrap	1 item (60 g)
		Pasta or rice	5 tablespoons (180 g)
		Breakfast cereal	1 bowl (40–50 g)
		Potatoes, sweet potatoes, yams	1 fist-sized (150 g)
3 Calcium-rich foods	2–4	*1 portion = 200 ml milk*	
		Milk (dairy or calcium-fortified soya milk)	1 medium cup (200 ml)
		Cheese	Size of 4 dice (40 g)
		Tofu	Size of 4 dice (60 g)
		Yoghurt/fromage frais	1 pot (150 ml)
4 Protein-rich foods	2–4	*1 portion = size of a deck of cards (70 g)*	
		Lean meat	3 slices

Food group	Number of portions each day	Food	Portion size
		Poultry	2 medium slices/ 1 chicken or turkey breast
		Fish	1 fillet (115–140 g)
		Eggs	2
		Lentils/beans	5 tablespoons (150 g)
		Tofu/soya burger or sausage	1–2
5 Healthy fats and oils	1–2	*1 portion = 1 tablespoon*	
		Nuts and seeds	2 tablespoons (25 g)
		Seed oils, nut oils	1 tablespoon (15 ml)
		Avocado	Half avocado
		Oily fish*	Deck of cards (140 g)
6 Foods and drinks high in sugars and/or fats	< 3	Biscuits	2
		Crisps	1 packet
		Chocolate	30 g (6 squares)
		Cereal bar	1 bar
		Cake	1 cupcake
		Sugary drink	500 ml

* Oily fish is very rich in essential fats so just 1 portion a week would cover a young athlete's needs

References

Boisseau, N. *et al.*, 'Protein Requirements in Male Adolescent Soccer Players', *European Journal of Applied Physiology*, May, 100(1) (2007), pp. 27–33.

Burke, D.G. *et al.*, 'Glycaemic Index – a New Tool in Sports Nutrition', *International Journal of Sport Nutrition*, 8 (1998), pp. 401–415.

Craig, W.J. *et al.*, 'Position of the American Dietetic Association: Vegetarian Diets', *Journal of the American Dietetic Association*, 109(7) (2009), pp. 1266–1282.

Department of Health, *Dietary Reference Values for Food Energy and Nutrients for the United Kingdom* (HMSO, 1991).

International Association of Athletic Federations (IAAF), *Nutrition for Athletics: The 2007 IAAF Consensus Statement* (IAAF, 2007).

International Olympic Committee (IOC), 'Consensus on Sports Nutrition, 2003', *Journal of Sports Science*, 22(1) (2003), p. x.

Lukaski, H.C., 'Vitamin and Mineral Status: Effects on Physical Performance', *Nutrition*, 20 (2004), pp. 632–644.

Macdougall, J.D. *et al.*, 'Maximal Aerobic Capacity of Canadian School Children: Prediction Based on Age-Related Oxygen Cost of Running', *Journal of Sports Medicine*, 4 (1982), pp. 194–198.

Phillips, S.M. *et al.*, 'A Critical Examination of Dietary Protein Requirements, Benefits and Excesses in Athletes', *International Journal of Sport Nutrition and Exercise Metabolism*, 17 (2007), pp. 58–78.

Rodriquez, N.R. *et al.*, 'Position of the American Dietetic Association, Dietitians of Canada, and the American College of Sports Medicine: Nutrition and Athletic Performance', *Journal of the American Dietetic Association*, 109(3) (2009), pp. 509–527.

Schofield, W.N. *et al.*, 'Basal Metabolic Rate – Review and Prediction', *Human Nutrition: Clinical Nutrition*, 39(suppl.) (1985), pp. 1–96.

Scientific Advisory Committee on Nutrition, *Salt and Health* (The Stationery Office, 2003).

Tarnopolsky, M., 'Building Muscle', Sport Nutrition Conference (Birmingham University, 2007).

Tipton, K. and Wolfe, R., 'Protein Needs and Amino Acids for Athletes', *Journal of Sports Science*, 22(1) (2007), pp. 65–79.

Wu, C.L. and Williams, C., 'A Low Glycaemic Index Meal Before Exercise Improves Endurance Running Capacity in Men', *Journal of Sports Nutrition and Exercise Metabolism*, 16 (2006), pp. 510–527.

02

EATING FOR SPORT

Eating the right type of food and drinking enough fluid before, during and after each training session will help young athletes perform better, reduce fatigue and prevent them getting ill.

This chapter will explain the key nutritional strategies that can be used to improve their training sessions. These centre around providing sufficient fuel for the muscles, maintaining hydration, and promoting post-exercise recovery. They can best be achieved by considering sports nutrition in three distinct phases:

1 before training;
2 during training;
3 after training.

This chapter will also provide some practical guidelines for pre-training meals, snacks and drinks; some suggestions for eating and drinking during training; and, finally, recommendations for what to eat and drink after training to promote fast recovery.

Before training

It's important that young athletes begin each training session fully fuelled and properly hydrated. This will allow them to exercise harder and for longer. Many studies have shown that a carbohydrate-rich diet before exercise results in increased endurance and better performance (e.g. Rodriquez, *et al.*, 2009). Conversely, an inadequate carbohydrate intake results in low muscle stores and reduced endurance. It increases the risk of early fatigue and poor performance. The athlete may struggle to keep up the pace, they may lag behind their teammates, they may feel weak, and they may have to stop training before the end of the session. It's rather like setting off in a car on a long journey with only half a tank of petrol. Without enough fuel, you won't be able to drive so far and you'll have to reduce your speed to conserve what little fuel you have. On the other hand, if you set off with plenty of fuel you'll be able to go faster and further.

WHAT IS THE PURPOSE OF THE PRE-EXERCISE MEAL?

The pre-exercise meal should provide the athlete with sustained energy, stop them feeling hungry during training, and be easily digested.

When should young athletes eat before training?

The optimal time for the pre-exercise meal is two to four hours before exercise (Hargreaves *et al.*, 2004). Carbohydrate in this meal will help top up muscle and liver glycogen levels and enhance performance during training or competition. If young athletes leave a longer gap than four hours, then they will almost certainly feel hungry during training, tired and light-headed. On the other hand, if they eat too much too close to training, then they may feel uncomfortable, 'heavy' or nauseous, and unable to train hard as the blood supply diverts to the digestive organs instead of the muscles.

In practice, the exact timing of their pre-exercise meal will probably depend on constraints such as school hours, travel, homework and training session times. Try to plan meals as best you can around these commitments. If the training session starts at 7 o'clock, plan to eat at about 5 o'clock. But if the athlete must train earlier, then they should eat a smaller meal, which is easier to digest, and which will produce the same benefits. They should feel comfortable, neither full nor hungry.

If the young athlete has to train straight after school, during their lunch break or first thing in the morning, then they may not have time for a meal. Instead, they should have a smaller meal or healthy snack, and include a drink. The food eaten should be easily digestible – high in carbohydrate, low in fat – such as toast, a cereal bar or a juice drink (*see* the box entitled 'Pre-training snacks' for more ideas).

What should young athletes eat before training?

The pre-training meal should be based on a high-carbohydrate food such as bread, pasta, potatoes or rice. These foods have a low glycaemic index (GI, *see* the box entitled 'What is the glycaemic index?'), which means they produce a gradual increase in blood sugar levels and give sustained energy. Studies have shown that athletes are able to exercise considerably longer after eating a low-GI meal compared with a high-GI meal (Chryssanthopoulos *et al.*, 2002). A low-GI meal helps maintain blood sugar levels, increase endurance and delay fatigue.

Include some protein in the pre-training meal: chicken, fish, cheese, egg, beans, lentils or nuts. This will assist in lowering the overall GI of the meal as well as help reduce muscle breakdown during exercise and improve performance (Kerksick *et al.*, 2008). Avoid too much fat as this takes longer to digest and may make the athlete feel uncomfortable during training. Fried foods, sausages, burgers and chips should be off the menu before training!

Porridge, cereal with milk, a jacket potato with beans or a light pasta meal would be suitable pre-workout meals (*see* the box entitled 'Pre-training meals' for more suggestions).

PRE-TRAINING MEALS

- Jacket potato with cheese, tuna or baked beans, plus salad
- Pasta with tomato-based sauce or pesto, a little cheese and some vegetables
- Rice, pasta or noodles with chicken, fish or beans, and vegetables
- A bowl of wholegrain breakfast cereal with milk and banana
- Porridge with milk, honey and raisins
- Lentil/vegetable or chicken soup with wholemeal bread
- Wholemeal sandwich/roll/wrap filled with tuna/cheese/chicken/peanut butter and salad

PRE-TRAINING SNACKS

If there is not time for a meal, the young athlete should have a snack 30 minutes before training, with a drink of water.

- One or two bananas (or other fresh fruit)
- A handful of dried fruit and nuts
- One or two cereal bars
- A pot of fruit yoghurt and some fresh fruit
- One or two slices of bread or toast with honey
- Two or three mini-pancakes
- A smoothie (home-made or ready bought)
- Rice cakes with peanut butter or a little cheese

WHAT IS THE GLYCAEMIC INDEX?

The glycaemic index (GI) is a ranking of foods from 0 to 100 based on their immediate effect on blood sugar levels. Glucose has a GI of 100. It's a measure of how quickly the food turns into glucose in the bloodstream. Foods with a high GI (above 70) cause a rapid rise in blood sugar levels. These include many refined ('white') starchy foods – such as cornflakes, white bread and white rice – as well as sugary foods such as soft drinks, biscuits and sweets.

Foods with a low GI (below 55) produce a slower and smaller blood sugar rise. These include beans, lentils, coarse-grain breads, muesli, fresh fruit and dairy products. Foods that contain no carbohydrate – meat, fish, chicken, eggs, oil, butter and margarine – have no GI value.

Table 2.1 lists examples of low-, medium- and high-GI foods.

Table 2.1 Low-, medium- and high-GI foods

Low-GI foods	Medium-GI foods	High-GI foods
Pasta	Brown and basmati rice	White bread and rolls, French bread and bagels
Beans and lentils	Pizza	Most breakfast cereals, e.g. cornflakes, Rice Krispies, Coco Pops
Milk and yoghurt	Chapatti	White rice

Low-GI foods	Medium-GI foods	High-GI foods
Peas	Pitta bread	Most wholemeal bread
Most vegetables, e.g. cucumber, broccoli	Boiled potatoes	Mashed and baked potatoes
		Doughnuts
Most fresh fruit, e.g. apples, pears, bananas, grapes, kiwi fruit	Tinned fruit	Chips
Dried apricots	Ice cream	Jam and sugar
Nuts	Raisins	Soft drinks
Porridge, bran cereals and muesli	Cereal bars	Sweets
Multigrain bread (e.g. granary)	Digestive biscuits	Most biscuits

Can sugar provide a pre-exercise energy boost?

I see lots of young athletes consuming sugary foods and drinks just before training, in the belief that the sugar in these products will help them train harder and longer. Although sugar is a fuel, eating too much of it can cause rapid fluctuations in blood sugar levels and, ironically, make athletes feel more tired. Sugar-rich foods and drinks produce a rapid rise in blood sugar levels, which in turn triggers the release of insulin to remove sugar from the bloodstream. Lots of sugar makes the body produce lots of insulin, which can result in low blood sugar levels, light-headedness, nausea and early fatigue during exercise. Rather than giving them extra energy, sugar may sap their energy!

They should avoid this by consuming only small amounts of sugar before exercise – less than 25 g generally produces a moderate increase in blood sugar – or opting for a food or drink with a lower GI. If they need a pre-training energy boost, it's safer to choose foods such as bananas, dried fruit and cereal bars that won't play havoc with blood sugar levels.

IF YOUNG ATHLETES HAVE TO TRAIN FIRST THING IN THE MORNING BUT DON'T FEEL HUNGRY, SHOULD THEY FORCE THEMSELVES TO EAT?

This is a bit of a dilemma because it is hard to make yourself eat when you aren't hungry, yet eating something will give the young athlete more energy for training, increase their endurance and help them perform better! However, it is possible to overcome an early-morning lack of appetite. First, they should avoid eating a big meal the night before as this takes a long time to digest fully. Second, see if they can manage just a few bites of food and a drink of water. They probably won't have time for a big breakfast, but a small healthy snack will make a big difference to their performance. They could try a cereal bar, a slice of toast, a small bowl of cereal, a couple of mini-pancakes or a banana. They should always have a drink – water is the best choice. They will have lost a lot of fluid in the night and will need to rehydrate before training.

If they really cannot face food first thing, they should have a nutritious drink, such as fruit juice, a smoothie, a milk-based drink (such as a milkshake or hot chocolate) or yoghurt drink. This will provide energy to fuel their muscles during training.

Get them to persevere – they will soon get used to the feeling of food and drink in their stomach early in the morning. And they will find that they'll be able to train harder and for longer.

What should young athletes drink before training?

It's important that young athletes are fully hydrated before they start training. They will have a better chance of putting in a good performance. If they are not properly hydrated before exercise, then they risk becoming more dehydrated during the training session and suffering early fatigue. Exercise will feel much harder than usual, they will tire quicker, and they risk dehydration symptoms, such as headaches, nausea and dizziness.

Prevention is better than cure. If they train in the evening, make sure they drink plenty of water during the day. If they train early in the morning, they should have a drink as soon as they get up. They will know if they are properly hydrated from the colour of their urine. It should be pale straw-coloured, not deep yellow, and should not have a strong odour. Try to get them into the habit of self-monitoring their hydration status. The 'pee chart' presented in Figure 2.1 provides a guide to hydration levels.

Encourage young athletes to make up for any previously incurred fluid deficits by consuming 400–600 ml about two hours before training or competition, and to continue drinking little and often during the warm-up.

When it comes to choosing what to drink, water is one of the best ways of hydrating the body. It is rapidly absorbed – and free too. Should they opt for a sports drink? Perhaps if they haven't eaten anything – in which case the sugars in the drink will help maintain blood sugar levels and fuel the muscles. Otherwise, water is a perfectly good pre-exercise choice, together with a pre-exercise meal or snack.

Figure 2.1 Urine chart

How much should young athletes drink each day?

There are no official guidelines for fluid intake, although many health professionals advise drinking 1.5 litres per day as a general guide (see the British Dietetic Association (BDA) and National Health Service (NHS) web pages listed in the 'References' section at the end of this chapter). The European Food Safety Authority (EFSA) recommends that children aged 9–13 years drink 1.3–1.5 litres daily; those over 14 years between 1.4 and 1.8 litres.

These recommendations don't take account of exercise, however. Young athletes will lose extra fluid through sweating during training, more in hot and humid conditions, and will certainly need to drink more than non-active people. They should drink little and often throughout the day rather than lots of water in one go. They must not ignore thirst, no matter how busy they are. The best way to tell whether they are drinking enough is from the colour of their urine (Figure 2.1). If it is yellow and has a strong odour (4 or above on the pee chart), they are dehydrated and need to drink more. It should always have a colour between 1 and 3 before they begin training.

Is it a good idea to have an energy drink before training?

Energy drinks have become increasingly popular among young athletes, who see them as an easy way to boost their performance. The clever marketing behind energy drinks suggests that they make you feel energetic. In fact, the opposite may be true! The term 'energy' refers to the drink's high energy (or calorie) content, not its ability to boost performance. Energy drinks comprise sugar and water. The sugar content is around 10–12 g per 100 g, or 25–31 g per 250 ml can, about the same concentration as most fizzy drinks, but too concentrated for the body to absorb quickly. At such high sugar concentrations, the fluid is absorbed more slowly from energy drinks compared with water or isotonic sports drinks, which makes them an unsuitable choice for exercise. In the USA, the National Federation of State High School Associations cautions against energy drinks for hydration and warns of the potential risk of dehydration associated with them (NFHS, 2008).

Can energy drinks with caffeine enhance performance?

Many energy drinks contain caffeine (about 80 mg per 250 ml, equivalent to a cup of coffee), which is known for its ability to increase mental alertness as well as endurance performance. But don't assume that young athletes will perform better with a caffeine boost. While caffeine is considered safe for use by adults, there is little research supporting its safety and effectiveness in young athletes. High doses can also cause side-effects: an upset stomach, sleeplessness, dizziness, headaches and higher blood pressure. Everyone responds differently – young athletes may be very sensitive to caffeine so could end up feeling nauseous or suffering from 'caffeine jitters' at a time when they are already nervous and anxious. Like any drug, it can also cause dependence, which means that they need more and more to get the same effect and, if they suddenly stop taking it, they may develop withdrawal symptoms (headaches, tiredness and irritability). The negative effects can outweigh potential performance benefits.

During training

During exercise the muscles produce heat, which raises the body's core temperature. To avoid the core temperature increasing excessively, the body uses a system known as thermoregulation. Heat is transferred from the muscles to the blood and blood flow to the skin is increased so that heat can escape into the atmosphere. The production of sweat and its evaporation from the skin also helps keep the body core temperature stable.

The amount of fluid lost in sweat depends on the surrounding temperature and humidity, and the intensity and duration of exercise. The warmer and more humid the conditions, and the longer and harder they exercise, the more fluid young athletes lose. Replacing these fluid losses is particularly important to prevent dehydration and its associated dangers.

What are the signs of dehydration?

Thermoregulation is less efficient in young athletes compared with adults; they produce sweat less readily than adults and have a greater surface area to body weight ratio, so are more susceptible to dehydration.

Common symptoms of dehydration include lack of energy, nausea, early fatigue, headaches and inability to concentrate. More severe symptoms include dizziness, vomiting, disorientation and increasing weakness. Eventually this can lead to exhaustion, heat stroke and, in some cases, can be fatal. Even mild dehydration – a 2 per cent loss in body weight – can impair performance, reduce stamina and strength, and increase fatigue.

WARNING SIGNS OF DEHYDRATION

Early symptoms

- Unusually lacking in energy
- Fatiguing early during exercise
- Headache
- Feeling very hot
- Skin appears flushed, and feels cool and clammy
- Passing only small volumes of dark-coloured urine
- Nausea

Action: Stop exercising. Drink 100–200 ml water or sports drink every 10–15 minutes.

Advanced symptoms

- Severe headache
- Becomes dizzy or light-headed
- Appears disorientated
- Short of breath

Action: Stop exercising. Drink 100–200 ml sports drink every 10–15 minutes. Seek professional help.

What's the best way of preventing dehydration?

Prevention is certainly better than cure. Encourage young athletes to start drinking early during their training session – within the first 30 minutes – and to continue drinking at regular intervals. It takes 15–30 minutes for fluid to be absorbed into the bloodstream so athletes should not wait until they feel thirsty or experience symptoms of dehydration before they start drinking. For most people, thirst is not a reliable guide to fluid losses. They may be dehydrated by the time they feel thirsty.

Help young athletes plan their drinking strategy for each training session and competition. As a rule of thumb, they should aim to drink around 500 ml per hour – more in hot, humid weather or when exercising very strenuously. If they exercise for a shorter time or at a lower intensity, they can drink proportionally less as the risk of dehydration will be smaller. Encourage them to drink little and often during training, ideally every 15–20 minutes or whenever there is an appropriate break. Make sure they have a water bottle (or two for longer sessions) and keep it within easy reach throughout training.

To get a more accurate idea of their fluid losses, young athletes can weigh them-selves before and after training. The American College of Sports Medicine recom-

IS IT HEALTHY TO DRINK MILK AFTER TRAINING?

There's growing evidence which suggests that milk may be just as effective as commercial sports drinks in helping athletes recover and rehydrate. It provides fluid for rehydration, as well as protein, vitamins and minerals such as calcium, potassium and magnesium that you need to replace after strenuous exercise. Milk's high content of protein and carbohydrate can help refuel exhausted muscles. The protein in milk helps build muscle tissue, and research suggests it may reduce exercise-induced muscle damage. A 2009 study from James Madison University, USA, found that chocolate milk promoted better muscle recovery compared with a commercial sports drink (Gilson *et al.*, 2009). Football players who drank chocolate milk after training had less muscle damage and faster muscle recovery compared with those who consumed a sports drink with the same amount of calories. Flavoured milk and plain milk have the advantage of additional nutrients not found in sports drinks and are therefore very good options as recovery drinks.

Refuelling snacks and drinks

Each of the following provides 50–60 g carbohydrate and 10–20 g protein. They should be consumed within two hours of exercise.

- 500 ml flavoured milk
- 1 banana plus 500 ml of milk
- 2 pots (2 x 150 g) of fruit yoghurt
- 1 cereal bar plus 500 ml semi-skimmed milk
- A smoothie – whizz 150 g yoghurt, 1 banana and 150 ml fruit juice in a blender
- A cheese sandwich (2 slices of bread, 40 g cheese)
- 60 g raisins and 50 g nuts
- 4 rice cakes with 20 g peanut butter plus 200 ml orange juice

REFUELLING MEALS

- Pasta with tomato sauce, grated cheese and vegetables
- Jacket potato, chicken breast, broccoli and carrots
- Bean and vegetable hotpot with wholegrain rice
- Rice with grilled fish and steamed vegetables
- Lasagne or vegetable lasagne with salad
- Fish pie with vegetables
- Chilli or vegetarian chilli with rice and vegetables
- Dahl (lentils) with rice and vegetables
- Chicken curry with rice and vegetables
- Mashed or baked potato with grilled salmon and salad

Menu plans

Use these menus as a basis for planning your daily menus. They have been designed to provide the optimum balance of protein, carbohydrate and fat, as well as fibre and essential vitamins and minerals, for young athletes. The menus supply approximately 2500 kcal, 3000 kcal and 3500 kcal to suit the energy needs of different individuals. There is also a plan for vegetarians. The quantities of each ingredient are listed, to show you how the daily nutritional analyses were calculated and also to give you an idea of how much food would be appropriate for young athletes. But it is not necessary to measure out their food so precisely every day! You may change the order of snacks and meals to suit individual training schedules. For more recipe ideas, *see* Chapter 6.

Menu for ... high-energy training (providing approximately 2500 calories)
Breakfast
Porridge made with 60 g oats, 300 ml skimmed milk, 1 tablespoon (20 g) of honey and 2 tablespoons (40 g) raisins

Snack
A serving (about 100 g) of fresh fruit
A cereal bar

Lunch
Wholemeal roll filled with tuna (50 g), mayonnaise (1 tablespoon) and cucumber
2 pots (2 x 150 g) fruit yoghurt
A serving (about 100 g) of fresh fruit

Pre-training snack (or afternoon snack)
A banana
A small handful (25 g) of nuts

During training
500 ml fruit juice mixed with 500 ml water

Post-training snack
300 ml flavoured milk

Supper
Chicken and vegetable stir-fry (*see* recipe, page 120)
Boiled rice (85 g uncooked weight)

Nutrition
2550 kcal
116 g protein
66 g fat (17 g saturates)
398 g carbohydrate

Menu for ... high-energy training (providing approximately 3000 calories)
Breakfast
2 slices wholegrain toast with margarine (20 g) and 1 tablespoon (20 g) of honey
A serving (about 100 g) of fresh fruit

Snack
1 (80 g) home-made or ready-bought flapjack (*see* recipe for honey flapjack, page 142)

Lunch
A wholemeal pitta (75 g) filled with cooked turkey (130 g), salad and a tablespoon (20 g) of mayonnaise
Yoghurt drink
A serving (about 100 g) of fresh fruit

Pre-training snack (or afternoon snack)
3 mini-pancakes with 1 tablespoon (20 g) of honey
A small handful of nuts (25 g)

During training
500 ml fruit juice mixed with 500 ml water

Post-training snack
A pot of yoghurt (150 g) and about 6 ready-to-eat dried apricots (120 g)

Supper
2 generous slices of pizza (400 g; *see* recipe, page 123), with salad or vegetables
Rice pudding (170 g; ready bought or home-made, *see* recipe page 139)

Nutrition
3058 kcal
123 g protein
90 g fat (26 g saturates)
468 g carbohydrate

Menu for ... high-energy training (providing approximately 3500 kcal)
Breakfast
2 poached eggs with 3 slices wholemeal toast and margarine (15 g)
A serving (about 100 g) of fresh fruit

Snack
A small handful of nuts (25 g) and raisins (60 g)

Lunch
2 wholemeal wraps filled with cooked chicken (80 g), 1 tablespoon (30 g) mayonnaise
and salad
A pot (150 g) of fruit yoghurt
A serving (about 100 g) of fresh fruit

Pre-training snack (or afternoon snack)
5 rice cakes with 1 tablespoon (30 g) peanut butter

During training
500 ml fruit juice diluted with 500 ml water

Post-training snack
300 ml semi-skimmed milk
2 cereal bars

Supper
2 jacket potatoes (400 g) with margarine (10 g)
Grilled plaice or other white fish (150 g) with vegetables or salad
2 bananas with a pot (150 g) of fruit yoghurt

Nutrition
3508 kcal
156 g protein
117 g fat (28 g saturates)
488 g carbohydrate

Menu for … vegetarians

Breakfast
Porridge made with oats (70 g) and 300 ml skimmed milk, a sliced banana and a tablespoon (20 g) of honey
A serving (about 100 g) of fresh fruit

Snack
A handful of nuts (40 g) and about 6 (120 g) ready-to-eat dried apricots

Lunch
Wholemeal pitta bread (75 g) filled with 2 tablespoons (50 g) grated cheese, grated carrot and a little (20 g) mayonnaise or salad cream
A pot of yoghurt (150 g)
Cherry tomatoes
A serving (about 100 g) of fresh fruit

Pre-training snack (or afternoon snack)
3 rice cakes with 1 tablespoon peanut butter

During training
500 ml fruit juice mixed with 500 ml water

Post-training snack
500 ml flavoured milk or low-fat milkshake

Supper
Macaroni cheese (200 g) with vegetables (*see* recipe, page 124)
A serving of strawberries or other fresh fruit (approx 100 g) with a pot (150 g) of fruit yoghurt

Nutrition
3048 kcal
115 g protein
99 g fat (28 g saturates)
453 g carbohydrate

References

ACSM, 'Exercise and Fluid Replacement', *Medicine & Science in Sports & Exercise*, 39 (2007), pp. 377–390.

Betts, J. *et al.*, 'The Influence of Carbohydrate and Protein Ingestion During Recovery from Prolonged Exercise on Subsequent Endurance Performance', *Journal of Sports Science*, 25(13) (2007), pp. 1449–1460.

Chryssanthopoulos, C. *et al.*, 'The Effect of a High Carbohydrate Meal on Endurance Running Capacity', *International Journal of Sport Nutrition*, 12, (2002), pp. 157–71.

Cockburn, E. *et al.*, 'Acute Milk-Based Protein-CHO Supplementation Attenuates Exercise-Induced Muscle Damage', *Applied Physiology, Nutrition, and Metabolism*, 33(4) (2008), pp. 775–783.

Coyle, E., 'Fluid and Fuel Intake During Exercise', *Journal of Sports Science*, 22 (2004), pp. 39–55.

Gilson, S.F. *et al.*, 'Effects of Chocolate Milk Consumption on Markers of Muscle Recovery During Intensified Soccer Training', *Medicine & Science in Sports & Exercise*, 41 (2009), p. S577

Gisolfi, C.V. *et al.*, 'Effect of Sodium Concentration in a Carbohydrate-Electrolyte Solution on Intestinal Absorption', *Med. Sci. Sports Ex.*, 27(10) (1995), pp. 1414–1420.

Hargreaves, M. *et al.*, 'Pre-Exercise Carbohydrate and Fat Ingestion: Effects on Metabolism and Performance', *Journal of Sports Science*, 22(1) (2004), pp. 31–38.

International Association of Athletic Federations (IAAF), *Nutrition for Athletics: The 2007 IAAF Consensus Statement* (IAAF, 2007).

International Olympic Committee (IOC), 'Consensus on Sports Nutrition, 2003', *Journal of Sports Science*, 22(1) (2004), p. x.

Ivy, J.L. *et al.*, 'Muscle Glycogen Synthesis After Exercise: Effect of Time of Carbohydrate Ingestion', *Journal of Applied Physiology*, 64 (1988), pp. 1480–1485.

Jeukendrup, A., 'Carbohydrate Intake During Exercise and Performance', *Nutrition*, 20 (2004), pp. 669–677.

Kerksick, C. *et al.*, 'International Society of Sports Nutrition Position Stand: Nutrient Timing', *Journal of the International Society of Sports Nutrition*, 3(5) (2008), p. 17.

Maughan, R.J. *et al.*, 'Rehydration and Recovery After Exercise', *Sports Sci. Ex.*, 9(62) (1996), pp. 1–5.

Maughan, R.J. & Leiper, J.B., 'Sodium intake and post-exercise rehydration in man', *European Journal of Applied Physiology*; 71(4):311-9.

National Federation of State High School Associations (NFSH), *Position Statement and Recommendations for the Use of Energy Drinks by Young Athletes* (NFSH, 2008).

Passe, D.H. *et al.*, 'Palatability and Voluntary Intake of Sports Beverages, Diluted Orange Juice and Water During Exercise', *International Journal of Sport Nutrition and Exercise Metabolism*, 14 (2004), pp. 272–284.

Rodriquez, N.R., Di Marco, N.M. and Langley, S., 'American College of Sports Medicine Position Stand: Nutrition and Athletic Performance. American Dietetic Association; Dietitians of Canada; American College of Sports Medicine', *Med Sci Sports Ex.*, 41(3) (2009), pp. 709–731.

Shireffs, S.M. *et al.*, 'Milk as an Effective Post-Exercise Rehydration Drink', *British Journal of Nutrition*, 98 (2007), pp. 173–180.

Tarnopolsky, M. and MacLennan, D.P., 'Post Exercise Protein-Carbohydrate and Carbohydrate Supplements Increase Muscle Glycogen in Males and Females', *Journal of Applied Physiology* (Abstracts), 4 (1997), p. 332A.

Van Loon, L.J.C., 'Application of Protein or Protein Hydrolysates to Improve Post-exercise Recovery', *Applied Physiology, Nutrition, and Metabolism*, 17 (2007), pp. S104–117.

Zawadski, K.M. *et al.*, 'Carbohydrate-protein complex increases the rate of muscle glycogen storage after exercise', *Journal of Applied Physiology* (1992), vol. 72, pp.1854-9.

03

WEIGHT AND SPORTS PERFORMANCE

For many sports, a low body fat percentage is associated with improved performance, but for children and adolescents there is not necessarily a linear relationship between the two. The issue of body weight and body fat percentage should be treated sensitively as misguided remarks or advice to young athletes may inadvertently result in an unhealthy obsession about their weight, body shape and food generally.

Clearly, young athletes who are a healthy weight for their build should not be encouraged to lose weight. If they are unhappy about their weight, the problem may be one of low self-esteem or being ill matched to their sport. For example, children with a larger build would not be well matched to thin-build sports such as distance running, gymnastics or ballet dancing.

The question as to whether overweight young athletes should be encouraged to lose weight is a tricky one and this should be discussed with a health professional. Much depends on their age, development stage, current weight and motivating reasons for losing weight.

This chapter considers the implications of weight loss for young athletes. These can be both positive and negative, so it is essential that any decision to lose weight should be made with professional guidance. This chapter also provides sensible strategies for achieving weight loss as well as weight gain.

Is there a link between a young athlete's weight, body fat percentage and performance?

Leanness is generally associated with better performance for virtually all sports. Excess body fat hinders performance: it reduces speed, agility, balance and endurance. Even for activities where a high body weight is advantageous for generating momentum, such as throwing, those athletes with a higher lean body mass percentage and lower fat percentage perform better.

But it is crucial to understand that there is no 'ideal' body fat percentage for young athletes. While improved performance is generally associated with lower-than-average body fat levels for many sports, there is certainly not a linear relationship between performance and body fat percentage. In other words, lower body fat levels are not always better. For each person, there is a range of body fat percentages at which they will perform at their best, and outside of which their performance and health are likely to suffer. Young athletes should not be put under pressure to attain an unrealistic low body weight and body fat percentage. Being lean does not guarantee athletic success.

Should overweight young athletes be encouraged to lose weight?

Any decision to lose weight should be made with the advice of a professional – such as a doctor, nutritionist or dietitian. Nutritional needs during this time are particularly high and important nutrients that are essential to children's health could be missed out.

Often, young athletes feel under pressure to lose weight to improve their performance and/or improve their appearance. They may see the successes of leaner competitors and be tempted to lose weight. Or they may feel frustrated by recent poor performance and perceive their weight to be the limiting factor for success in their sport. Sometimes, a decision to embark on a weight-loss regime may be triggered by a careless remark made by a well-meaning coach or teammate. The problem is that, without proper help, a desire to lose weight may develop into obsessive eating and exercise behaviour that could put their performance and health at risk. In such cases, young athletes, whether overweight or not, should be discouraged from losing weight. Instead, parents and coaches should try to build the young athlete's self-esteem and help them feel more positive about their weight and performance. Praising their successes and emphasising their strengths should help reduce undue anxiety about their weight.

On the other hand, for young athletes who are genuinely overweight, losing a few pounds through sensible eating and increased activity is likely to have a positive impact on their performance and health. It is important that they receive accurate information about nutrition, and positive support from their coach, family and friends.

How can I evaluate a young athlete's weight?

It can be difficult to evaluate whether young athletes have a weight problem. As a starting point, you can calculate their body mass index (BMI) – their weight in kg divided by the square of their height in metres – and compare with the children's BMI-for-age charts published by the US Centres for Disease Control and Prevention (CDC) (*see* http://www.cdc.gov/healthyweight/assessing/bmi/index.html). This will tell you whether their body weight is higher than average for their height and age. Table 3.1 gives the BMIs for overweight and obese children.

But BMI is not perfect. For example, it's very common for children to gain weight quickly – and for their BMI to go up – during puberty. They can also have a high BMI if they have a large frame or a lot of muscle, not excess fat. BMI does not differentiate between muscle and fat so it can be misleading when used with young athletes. Many of the world's top athletes have high BMIs due to their high muscularity, which would classify them as overweight. Thus, a young athlete who is relatively heavy due to a high muscle mass may have a high BMI for his or her age, and a child with a small frame may have a normal BMI but too much body fat.

It's important to look at the BMI values as a trend instead of focusing on individual numbers. Any one measurement, taken out of context, can give you the wrong impression of a young athlete's growth. The real value of BMI measurements lies in viewing them as a pattern over time. This allows doctors and parents to watch a child's growth and determine whether it is normal compared with that of other children of the same age.

To determine whether they have excess fat, further assessment would be needed. This might include bioelectrical impedance or skinfold thickness measurements.

Table 3.1 BMIs for overweight and obese children

Age	Overweight		Obese	
	Boys	**Girls**	**Boys**	**Girls**
5	17.4	17.1	19.3	19.2
6	17.6	17.3	19.8	19.7
7	17.9	17.8	20.6	20.5
8	18.4	18.3	21.6	21.6
9	19.1	19.1	22.8	22.8
10	19.8	19.9	24.0	24.1
11	20.6	20.7	25.1	25.4
12	21.2	21.7	26.0	26.7
13	21.9	22.6	26.8	27.8

Source: Cole *et al.* (2000)

How can I measure body fat percentage in young athletes?

Body fat levels in children and adolescents can be estimated using bioelectrical impedance or skinfold thickness measurements.

Bioelectrical impedance

This is the principle used in body composition analysers and body fat scales, widely available in shops and gyms. Many are calibrated for different ages and both genders, and are suitable for use with young athletes (Phillips *et al.*, 2003). A mild electrical current (completely painless!) is sent through the body, either from foot to foot or foot to opposite hand. The current passes more easily and more quickly through lean mass, but much more slowly through fat mass. The more body fat present, the greater the resistance. This method is less accurate for very lean and very overweight people.

Skinfold thickness

This method is widely used in sports clubs and has been shown to provide an accurate estimate of body fat percentage in children and adolescents (Deurenberg, 1990). The callipers measure the thickness of the layer of fat beneath the skin at various sites of the body. It works on the theory that 50 per cent of the total body fat is stored under the skin. Most assessments involve measurements at four sites: the triceps, biceps, below the shoulder blades, and midway between the hip and navel. The accuracy depends on the level of skill of the person taking the measurements. It is less accurate for very lean and obese individuals.

Don't snack-and-view

Discourage eating meals or unhealthy snacks while watching television. Because their mind will be on the television and not on the food, they won't notice when they are full up or not hungry any more.

Top tips for maintaining a healthy weight

The following strategies will make it easier for young athletes to achieve a healthy weight.

- They should eat foods that fill them up, not out – starting a meal with a bowl of soup, a salad, some fresh fruit or some fresh vegetables helps take the edge of hunger pangs. People who follow this eating pattern feel more satisfied at the end of a meal and consume fewer calories.
- Ditch the fizz – drinking water rather than sugary fizzy drinks is a good way of saving calories, and water won't rot their teeth or leach calcium from their bones.
- Follow the one-third rule – vegetables or salad should fill at least one-third of the plate. This will help satisfy hunger as well as providing essential nutrients.
- They should always eat food sitting at a table – eating in front of the TV or eating on the run makes people eat more because they don't concentrate fully.
- They should never skip meals – no matter how busy they are. Leaving gaps longer than four hours between meals not only saps energy but also triggers muscle loss, as

the body turns to protein for fuel. Young athletes should eat three small meals spread over the day – breakfast, lunch and evening meal – with two healthy snacks in between. Small, regular meals keep the metabolism revved up so that more calories are burned off each day.

■ Replace full-fat dairy products with low-fat varieties – they contain just as much protein and calcium.

■ They should opt for brown instead of white – wholegrain bread, bran cereals and whole-wheat pasta are rich in fibre, which will make them feel fuller. They should make the switch gradually, though, to avoid stomach upsets.

■ Make sure they don't wolf down their food – eating food slowly and in a relaxed state of mind will curb the desire to eat more then they need. According to research, scoffing a meal means that the satiety centre in the brain doesn't receive the right signals, and explains why people may eat more than they need.

■ They should start the day with a healthy breakfast, such as porridge. People who skip breakfast to 'save calories' are more likely to overeat later in the day and pile on unwanted pounds.

■ Get them to eat until they are satisfied, not stuffed. They should eat when they are truly hungry and stop when they feel satisfied, and avoid eating to the point where they feel stuffed and uncomfortable. By eating a bit slower, the brain has more time to get the 'full up' message.

■ They should avoid mindless munching – help them to find another distraction, or eat something that's low in calories, such as carrot sticks or apple slices.

Can young athletes be too thin?

If you are worried about a young athlete being too thin, it's important to understand that many children who weigh less than others their age are perfectly healthy. They may go through puberty later than some of their peers, and their bodies may grow and change at a different rate. Most underweight teens catch up in weight as they finish puberty during their later teen years, and there's rarely a need to try to gain weight.

In a few cases, young athletes can be underweight because of a health problem. If they feel tired or are ill frequently, or have symptoms such as a cough, stomach ache, diarrhoea or other problems that have lasted for more than a week or two, seek the advice of your doctor.

Some young athletes are underweight because of eating disorders, like anorexia or bulimia, that require attention. The pressure to be thin or attain better performance may trigger unhealthy eating behaviours that put their health at risk. It has been estimated that up to 60 per cent of female athletes suffer from disordered eating (Sundgot-Borgen, 1994). It appears to be more common in athletes involved in 'thin-build' sports, where a low body weight, low body fat percentage or thin build is perceived to be advantageous (Beals and Manore, 2002). These can be considered in four categories, as shown in Table 3.2.

How can young athletes increase muscle mass?
Training
To add muscle mass, their muscles need a stimulus to get bigger and stronger, and that requires a well-designed resistance training programme. Previous beliefs that resistance training can damage the growth cartilage or stunt their growth have proven to be unfounded – there have been no cases of bone damage in relation to resistance training. Exercises that emphasise strengthening of the core are recommended for pre-adolescent and adolescent children. Only after they have passed puberty should they consider adding muscle bulk. The best guidance comes from the American Academy of Paediatrics Committee on Sports Medicine and Fitness. Here is a summary of its updated policy statement (American Academy of Paediatrics, 2008):

- *Strength training programs for pre-adolescents and adolescents can be safe and effective if proper resistance training techniques and safety precautions are followed.*
- *Pre-adolescents and adolescents should avoid competitive weight lifting, power lifting, body building, and maximal lifts until they reach physical and skeletal maturity.*
- *Before beginning a formal strength training program, a medical evaluation should be performed. If indicated, a referral may be made to a sports medicine specialist who is familiar with various strength training methods as well as risks and benefits in pre-adolescents and adolescents.*
- *Aerobic conditioning should be coupled with resistance training if general health benefits are the goal.*
- *Strength training programs should include a warm-up and cool-down component.*
- *Specific strength training exercises should be learned initially with no load (resistance). Once the exercise skill has been mastered, incremental loads can be added.*
- *Progressive resistance exercise requires the successful completion of 8 to 15 repetitions in good form before increasing weight or resistance.*
- *A general strengthening program should address all major muscle groups and exercise through the complete range of motion.*
- *Any sign of injury or illness from strength training should be evaluated before continuing the exercise in question.*

Nutrition
The nutritional part of the equation for adding muscle mass is consuming adequate energy and nutrients, with energy perhaps being the most important. When it comes to adding muscle, many young (and also adult) athletes make the mistake of focusing solely on protein intake. To put on muscle, they need to consume about 500 more calories than they burn each day. They do need a little extra protein but most can get this from a balanced diet. In fact, the timing of their protein intake in relation to workouts is just as important as the amount.

Resistance training increases the rate at which muscle protein is made after a training session. So encourage young athletes to consume around 10–20 g protein within 30 minutes of training and as part of their protein–carbohydrate recovery snack (*see* Chapter 2, page 55, 'What should young athletes eat after training?'). This will help repair muscle tissue damaged during training, and support the making of new muscle tissue proteins. The meal or snack should contain about four times as much carbohydrate as protein. Good options include low-fat milk, flavoured milk, yoghurt, yoghurt drinks or home-made milkshakes (*see* page 57, 'Refuelling snacks and drinks').

HIGH-ENERGY SNACKS FOR WEIGHT GAIN

- Nuts – peanuts, almonds, cashews, brazils, pistachios
- Dried fruit – raisins, sultanas, apricots, dates
- Sandwiches, rolls, wraps and bagels filled with cheese, chicken, ham, tuna, peanut butter or banana
- Yoghurt
- Milk, milkshakes, flavoured milk, yoghurt drinks
- Breakfast cereal or porridge with milk
- Cheese
- Cheese on toast
- Mini-pancakes, scones, fruit buns, malt loaf
- Cereal bars
- Bread or toast with jam or honey

References

American Academy of Pediatrics, 'Strength Training by Children and Adolescents', *Pediatrics*, 121(4) (2008), pp. 835–840.

Beals, K.A. and Manore, M.M., 'Disorders of the Female Athlete Triad Among Collegiate Athletes', *International Journal of Sport Nutrition and Exercise Metabolism*, 12 (2002), pp. 281–293.

Cole, T.J., Bellizzi, M., Flegal, K. and Dietz, W.H., 'Establishing a Standard Definition for Child Overweight and Obesity Worldwide: International Survey', *British Medical Journal*, 320 (2000), pp. 1240–1243.

Deurenberg, P., 'The Assessment of the Body Fat Percentage by Skinfold Thickness Measurements in Childhood and Young Adolescence', *British Journal of Nutrition*, 63 (1990), pp. 293–303.

Hulley, A.J. and Hill, A.J. 'Eating Disorders and Health in Elite Women Distance Runners', *International Journal of Eating Disorders*, 30(3) (2001), pp. 312–317.

Jebb, S., McCarthy, D., Fry, T. and Prentice, A.M., 'New Body Fat Reference Curves for Children', *Obesity Reviews* (NAASO suppl.) (2004), p. A146.

Phillips, S.M., Bandini, L.G., Compton, D.V., Naumova, E.N. and Must, A.A., 'Longitudinal Comparison of Body Composition by Total Body Water and Bioelectrical Impedance in Adolescent Girls', *Journal of Nutrition*, 133(5) (1 May, 2003), pp. 1419–1425.

Sundgot-Borgen, J., 'Eating Disorders in Female Athletes', *Sports Medicine*, 17(3) (1994), pp. 176–188.

Sundgot-Borgen, J. and Torstveit, M.K., 'Prevalence of Eating Disorders in Elite Athletes is Higher than in the General Population', *Clinical Journal of Sport Medicine*, 14(1) (2004), pp. 25–32.

NUTRITIONAL SUPPLEMENTS

In the quest to improve their performance and gain a competitive edge, many young athletes take nutritional supplements, often without really knowing what they are or how they work. A 2005 survey revealed that 62 per cent of UK junior national track and field athletes used them regularly (Nieper, 2005). Each athlete took an average of 2.4 supplements. Multivitamins and minerals were the most popular, but 17 different supplements were identified in the survey. In another study of adolescent German athletes, 80 per cent reported taking various supplements, including sports drinks and energy supplements (Braun *et al.*, 2009).

So do young athletes really need them? Are they likely to benefit or harm their performance? The fact that many adult athletes take supplements does not mean that they are safe or effective for children and adolescents. Currently, nutritional supplements are not regulated for safety, purity, potency or efficacy, and manufacturers do not have to demonstrate that they are safe for children. Supplements may contain impurities or interact with medicines, and there is a possibility that certain products may contain impurities that would cause a positive drugs test (Schänzer, 2002).

This chapter provides information and evidence about the most popular nutritional supplements, to help you make up your own mind.

Caffeine

Young athletes often take caffeine in the form of energy drinks, sports drinks or cola before and during training or competition, in the belief that it will enhance their endurance, performance, concentration, motivation and mental alertness, and mask fatigue.

So what exactly is caffeine? It is a stimulant and, strictly speaking, is classed as a drug rather than a nutritional supplement. It is found in many everyday drinks, such as coffee, black and green tea, and cola, as well as chocolate (cocoa), and some brands of sports drinks, energy drinks and gels.

Caffeine works by decreasing the perception of effort during exercise, therefore allowing the athlete to perform at a higher intensity. It boosts adrenaline levels, which increases the levels of fatty acids in the bloodstream and encourages the muscles to use more fatty acids instead of glucose or glycogen (carbohydrate) for fuel. In theory, at least, caffeine may help athletes exercise longer and harder.

There are no official UK guidelines on caffeine for children but a review undertaken by Health Canada scientists considers 85 mg per day safe for 10–12 year olds

(Health and Welfare Canada, 2003). Food Standards Australia New Zealand recommends that children consume less than 95 mg per day (FSANZ, 2000). High doses of caffeine (greater than 95 mg daily) greatly increase the risks of negative side-effects – nervousness, an upset stomach, difficulty sleeping, anxiety, rapid heartbeat, dizziness and headaches – in some individuals. This equates to a cup of coffee, two cups of tea, or approximately one (500 ml) caffeinated sports drink or one (250 ml) energy drink.

But the safety and effectiveness of consuming caffeine before and during exercise has yet to be established with children and teenage athletes. They may be extra sensitive to caffeine so could experience the negative side-effects more than adults and end up suffering from 'caffeine jitters' at a time when they are already nervous and anxious. The side-effects may outweigh the potential benefits of caffeine for performance.

It's also worth remembering that caffeine is a diuretic, which means that it causes the body to lose water through urination. While studies with adults suggest that regular, moderate caffeine intakes do not dehydrate the body, the effect of caffeinated sports drinks on hydration in young athletes remains unknown. High doses – equivalent to one or two sports drinks – or infrequent caffeine consumption may have a more noticeable diuretic effect in young athletes.

The bottom line is that there are still many unknowns about the effect of caffeine on the performance and health of young athletes. Until more research is done, caffeine cannot be recommended.

THE CAFFEINE CONTENT OF VARIOUS FOODS AND DRINKS

- Instant coffee – 60 mg/cup
- Espresso – 100 mg/shot
- Cafetiere/filter – 120 mg/cup
- Tea – 40 mg/cup
- Green tea – 40 mg/cup
- Sports drinks with caffeine (e.g. Lucozade Sport Caffeine Boost) – 80 mg/500 ml
- Energy drinks (e.g. Red Bull) – 80 mg/250 ml
- Cola – 40 mg/330 ml
- Energy gel – 25 mg/sachet
- Dark chocolate – 40 mg/50 g
- Milk chocolate – 12 mg/50 g

Creatine

Creatine is extremely popular with adult athletes, who use it for its purported performance-boosting and muscle-building effects. Although the use of creatine is not recommended in people less than 18 years of age, several reports indicate widespread use in young athletes (Metzi *et al.*, 2001).

Creatine is a protein that is made naturally in the body from three amino acids, but can also be found in meat and fish, or taken in higher doses as a supplement. It is most commonly taken as a powder mixed with water or within an 'all-in-one' protein and energy mix.

In the body it combines with phosphorus to form phosphocreatine (PC) in the muscle cells. This is an energy-rich compound that fuels the muscles during anaerobic activities, such as lifting weights, sprinting, jumping or throwing. The aim of creatine supplementation is to enhance the muscles' content of PC, which in turn would increase the amount of energy generated during brief periods of high-intensity exercise. Theoretically, it may allow athletes to sustain all-out effort longer than usual, recover faster between 'sets' of high-intensity exercise, and increase muscle mass and strength gains. Indeed, studies with adult athletes have suggested that creatine supplements can improve performance in high-intensity activities, as well as increase total and lean body weight (Volek and Kraemer, 1996). However, there have been some studies showing no effect of creatine supplementation on performance (Kreider, 2003). It doesn't work for some individuals and is also unlikely to benefit endurance performance.

Unfortunately, there is little information about creatine use or the potential health risk in children and adolescents. Whether it is effective or safe in the long term has not been established. It is worth considering that performance during childhood and adolescence tends to be limited by mechanical factors rather than the relative contribution of the aerobic and anaerobic energy systems. A review by US researchers published in the *Journal of Strength and Conditioning Research* concluded that there is not enough research to support the use of creatine supplements by children and adolescents (Unnithan *et al.*, 2001).

Until the safety of creatine can be established in adolescents, the use of this product should be discouraged.

Energy bars

Energy bars are rich in carbohydrates and claim to provide a good source of fuel before and during exercise. However, don't assume that they will make anyone feel more energetic – that's what the manufacturers would want you to believe! The name on the label actually refers to the bar's high energy (calorie) content per gram.

The main ingredients are sugars (glucose, corn syrup, fructose) and maltodextrins (a carbohydrate made from corn starch). Bars may also contain small amounts of soy or whey protein, oat bran or cereal. Typically, they provide between 200 and 250 calories and 40–45 g of carbohydrate per bar. The protein and fat content is usually low.

On the plus side, consuming an energy bar before exercise may help increase endurance and improve performance – but not necessarily more than other carbohydrate-rich foods. Manufacturers also claim that energy bars provide a sustained source of energy, due to their high content of maltodextrin, which is digested more slowly than sugars. This results in a slower increase in blood sugar levels, compared with glucose (i.e. a low glycaemic response), which studies suggest can help increase endurance performance (Thomas *et al.*, 1991). But other foods can provide a similar performance benefit. Suitable pre-exercise snacks include cereal bars, dried fruit, bananas, and rice cakes with peanut butter.

On the minus side, the cost of energy bars may be prohibitive for young athletes. Explain to them that energy bars are not necessarily better for their performance than other foods, that they can get similar benefits from cheaper foods. Be aware, too, of the energy (calorie) content of bars. Many brands contain the same number of calories as popular chocolate and confectionery bars, and may be more than the athlete is likely to burn during the activity session! Over-consuming calories may result in weight gain.

In conclusion, the main benefit of consuming an energy bar before or during exercise is convenience. They are portable and non-perishable but there is no reason why they represent a better snack option than other high-carbohydrate foods.

Energy gels

Energy gels are carbohydrate-rich, jelly-like supplements that come in small squeezy sachets and are designed to be consumed on the move during endurance exercise. Many athletes appreciate their convenience but you should also be aware of alternative ways of fuelling on the go.

Energy gels consist almost entirely of simple sugars (such as fructose and glucose) and maltodextrin (made from corn starch). Some brands also contain sodium, potassium and caffeine (*see* the section on caffeine, above). Most contain between 18 and 25 g of carbohydrate per sachet.

On the plus side, gels provide a convenient way of consuming carbohydrate during intense endurance exercise lasting longer than an hour. Their small size means that they can easily be stashed in pockets, opened with ease when running, for example, and consumed quickly in the manner of knocking back a 'shot'. They provide around 18–25 g of rapidly absorbed carbohydrate, which should fuel between 30 and 60 minutes of exercise. The scientific consensus is to consume 30–60 g of carbohydrate per hour during prolonged exercise in order to delay fatigue and improve endurance (Rodriquez *et al.*, 2009).

On the downside, some people dislike their texture, sweetness and intensity of flavour – it's really down to personal preference. Gels don't provide hydration so, if young athletes want to use them, encourage them to drink plenty of water at the same time. A handy rule of thumb would be to follow one sachet with 500 ml of water consumed over 60 minutes, or half a gel sachet followed by 250 ml of water over 30 minutes. If they don't drink enough, they could end up with stomach ache as the gel sits in their stomach. Drinking plenty of water effectively dilutes the gel, allowing the

Coyle, E., 'Fluid and Fuel Intake During Exercise', Journal of Sports Science, 22 (2004), pp. 39–55.

Food Standards Australia New Zealand (FSANZ), 'Report from the Expert Working Group on the Safety Aspects of Dietary Caffeine' (2000), http://www.food-standards.gov.au/.

Heath and Welfare Canada, 'Caffeine and Your Health' (2003), http://www.hc-sc.gc.ca/fn-an/securit/facts-faits/caffeine-eng.php.

International Association of Athletic Federations (IAAF) *Nutrition for Athletics: The 2007 IAAF Consensus Statement* (IAAF, 2007).

International Olympic Committee (IOC), 'Proceedings of a Consensus Conference of the International Olympic Committee Medical Commission Nutrition and Sport Working Group (15–18 June, 2003), Lausanne, Switzerland', *Journal of Sports Science*, 22(1) (2004), pp. vii–x; 1–145.

Kreider, R.B., 'Effects of Creatine Supplementation on Performance and Training Adaptations', *Mol. Cell. Biochem.*, 244 (2003), pp. 89–94.

Metzi, J.D. *et al.*, 'Creatine Use Among Young Athletes', *Pediatrics*, 108(2) (2001), pp. 421–425.

National Federation of State High School Associations (NFHS), *Position Statement and Recommendations for the Use of Energy Drinks by Young Athletes* (NFHS, 2008).

Nieper, A., 'Nutritional Supplement Practices in UK Junior National Track and Field Athletes', British Journal of Sports Medicine, 39(9) (2005), pp. 645–649.

Rodriquez, N.R., Di Marco, N.M. and Langley, S., 'American College of Sports Medicine Position Stand: Nutrition and Athletic Performance. American Dietetic Association; Dietitians of Canada; American College of Sports Medicine', *Med Sci Sports Ex.*, 41(3) (2009), pp. 709–731.

Schänzer, W., *Analysis of Non-Hormonal Nutritional Supplements for Anabolic-Androgenic Steroids – an International Study*, Institute of Biochemistry, German Sport University Cologne (2002), http://multimedia.olympic.org/pdf/en_report_324.pdf.

Thomas, D.E. *et al.*, 'Carbohydrate Feeding Before Exercise: Effect of Glycaemic Index', *International Journal of Sports Medicine*, 12 (2002), pp. 180–186.

Unnithan, V.B. *et al.*, 'Is There a Physiologic Basis for Creatine Use in Children and Adolescents?', *J. Strength Cond. Res.*, 15(4) (2001), pp. 524–8.

Volek, J.S. and Kraemer, W.J., 'Creatine Supplementation: Its Effects on Human Muscular Performance and Body Composition', *J. Strength Cond. Res.*, 10(3) (1996), pp. 200–210.

Walser, B. and Stebbins, C.L., 'Omega-3 Fatty Acid Supplementation Enhances Stroke Volume and Cardiac Output During Dynamic Exercise', *European Journal of Applied Physiology*, 104(3) (2008), pp. 455–461.

Walser, B., Giordano, R.M. and Stebbins, C.L., 'Supplementation with Omega-3 Polyunsaturated Fatty Acids Augments Brachial Artery Dilation and Blood Flow During Forearm Contraction', *European Journal of Applied Physiology*, 97(3) (2006), pp. 347–354.

05

EATING FOR COMPETITION

Competitions are an integral part of most sports. They provide a reason for young athletes to train, goals to aim for, and opportunities for them to put into practice the fitness and the skills they have developed after weeks and months of hard training.

Whether they are competing in a race, a match, or a tournament involving several events, young athletes need to be well prepared nutritionally. What they eat and drink in the days and hours before a competition, as well as during the competition, can make a big difference to their performance. If they arrive at the event properly fuelled and well hydrated, then they will have a competitive edge. But if they compete low on fuel and dehydrated, they will not put in their best performance. Planning ahead will help them have a successful competition and avoid food-related problems on the day. This chapter provides a nutrition guide to help young athletes prepare for competition.

The week before

During the last few days before a competition, young athletes should continue eating their normal diet. Make sure they stick to healthy eating principles as closely as possible during this time and that they stay well hydrated. They should focus on carbohydrate-rich foods in their diet – potatoes, pasta, rice and bread – to replenish glycogen levels after each training session, and drink plenty of water throughout the day. Encourage them to eat to their appetite – if they feel hungry, then provide bigger portions and healthy snacks, but do not 'force feed' them if they are not hungry.

There is no need to manipulate the energy or carbohydrate content of their diet. Young athletes do not need to carbohydrate-load (consume extra carbohydrates in the last few days before a competition) – this is appropriate only for experienced athletes competing in endurance events lasting longer than 90 minutes.

For bigger competitions, they should, if possible, taper their training for a few days. This may mean reducing their training time and resting for a day or two before the event. The idea is to give the muscles an opportunity to fully repair themselves, and to refuel after an intense training period.

For smaller competitions, most coaches do not consider a taper necessary, apart from perhaps easing the training intensity of the last session. If young athletes are expected to compete frequently, say once a week, then it may be considered disruptive to their training schedule to taper for each competition. However, individual judgement would dictate whether and when the young athlete takes a rest day.

Q: SHOULD YOUNG ATHLETES CARBOHYDRATE LOAD BEFORE COMPETITIONS?

A: Carbohydrate loading is a nutrition and training strategy designed to maximise muscle glycogen stores before endurance competitions. Originally devised in the 1960s, it used to involve a three-day depletion phase (hard training combined with a low carbohydrate intake) followed by a three-day loading phase (light training combined with a high carbohydrate intake). Nowadays, experts advise omitting the depletion phase, as this provides no benefit. Carbohydrate loading has been shown to improve endurance performance by 2–3 per cent in events lasting longer than 90 minutes, such as cycling, marathon running, longer-distance triathlon, cross-country skiing and long-distance swimming. But studies have been carried out only with adult men, not women, children or adolescent athletes, so it is not possible to say whether carbohydrate loading would work with young athletes. Given that few young athletes would be competing continually at a moderate or high intensity for longer than 90 minutes, carbohydrate loading is probably not a realistic option. For most sports, young athletes should aim to consume their usual diet prior to competition, perhaps increasing carbohydrate-rich foods and cutting down on high-fat foods during the last few days to facilitate glycogen storage.

Top tips for the week before a competition

- Stick to familiar foods and drinks – young athletes should not try anything new in the last few days in case it does not agree with them.
- Eat little and often – dividing their food into several small meals and snacks will make it easier to digest, keep their blood sugar levels steady and encourage muscle glycogen storage in preparation for the event.
- See that they don't skip meals – leaving long gaps between eating may result in low fuel stores before the competition.
- Ensure that they drink plenty of water – they need to keep well hydrated by drinking at least 1.5 litres a day, plus another 0.5 litres for each hour of exercise (they may need more in hot weather). Water is one of the healthiest options, but fruit juice, squash and milk also count.
- They should avoid overeating late in the evening – big meals before bedtime may make them feel uncomfortable and lethargic the next day.
- Choose slow-burn meals – eating carbohydrate with protein provides sustained energy for all-day fuelling. Suitable options include baked potato with beans, pasta with chicken, rice with fish.
- They should cut down on 'empty calories' – reducing their intake of foods high in saturated fats and added sugars, such as confectionery, pastries, crisps and fast foods, and instead eat nutrient-rich foods such as whole grains, fruit and vegetables which will prepare young athletes better for competition.

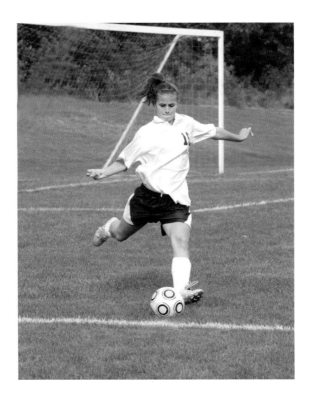

Test in training what they plan to do during the competition

Now is the time to rehearse their competition-day eating and drinking strategy. Whatever they plan to eat and drink during the competition should be rehearsed in training. They may experiment with different foods and drinks to find the types and amounts that suit them best. It's a good idea to research the foods and drinks to be provided at the venue so that you can plan what to take with you. Generally, it's safer to take your own supplies.

Eating on the move

Sometimes young athletes have to travel long distances to competitions, and spend hours in a car, coach, train or aeroplane. It's easy to forget to drink, and get dehydrated, so organise a travelling nutrition strategy.

Make sure they take their own supplies of food and drink for the journey. Do not rely on being able to find the right foods at outlets en route or at the venue – healthy choices are often limited at these places.

If they're travelling abroad, it's important to avoid common food-poisoning culprits – chicken, seafood and meat dishes – unless you're sure they have been properly cooked and heated to a high temperature. As a rule of thumb, avoid anything that is lukewarm. Also, peel fruit and veg, stick to bottled water and avoid ice in drinks.

Q: SHOULD YOUNG ATHLETES EAT ANYTHING BEFORE AN EARLY-MORNING START ON COMPETITION DAY?

A: Many young athletes don't feel like eating, and struggle to eat a pre-competition meal early in the morning, partly due to nerves, partly due to the early start. But it's crucial that they consume at least a small amount of carbohydrate to raise blood glucose levels and top up muscle glycogen stores following the overnight fast. Competing on empty may result in low blood glucose levels, light-headedness, nausea and a poor performance. If a meal is out of the question, they should try to have a nutritious snack, such as wholemeal toast with honey, a cereal bar or a banana. Alternatively, try them with a nutritious drink, such as milk, hot chocolate, flavoured milk, a smoothie or a milk-shake. Diluted juice or a sports drink would also be a suitable option, but steer them away from sweets, sugary drinks and energy drinks, which may have an unpredictable effect on their blood glucose level. Encourage them to drink water or diluted juice upon waking, and then to continue drinking little and often before competing.

Suitable foods for eating on the move include:

- sandwiches filled with peanut butter, banana, honey, chicken, tuna or cheese (keep in an insulated chiller bag if possible);
- rice cakes, oatcakes and wholemeal crackers;
- individual cheese portions;
- small bags of nuts – peanuts, cashews, almonds;

- fresh fruit – apples, bananas, grapes;
- dried fruit – apricots, raisins, mangoes;
- cereal bars;
- prepared vegetable crudités, e.g. tomatoes, carrots (keep in a chiller bag if possible).

Suitable drinks on the move include:

- bottles of water;
- cartons of fruit juice;
- yoghurt drinks;
- low-fat milk.

SUITABLE RESTAURANT MEALS AND FAST FOODS WHEN TRAVELLING TO A COMPETITION

- Simple pasta dishes with tomato sauce
- Plain rice with vegetables, chicken or fish
- Pizza with tomato and vegetable toppings
- Simple noodle dishes (not fried)
- Jacket potatoes with beans, tuna or cheese

RESTAURANT MEALS AND FAST FOODS TO AVOID

- Anything deep-fried
- Burgers and chips
- Chicken nuggets
- Pasta with creamy or oily sauces
- Takeaway curries
- Takeaway kebabs
- Battered fish and chips
- Hot dogs
- Fried chicken meals

Q: ARE CAFFEINE-CONTAINING ENERGY DRINKS SUITABLE FOR YOUNG ATHLETES DURING COMPETITION?

A: Many young athletes use caffeine-containing energy drinks before and during competition, in the belief that these drinks will give them a performance advantage. However, a 2009 review of health claims by the European Food Safety Authority (EFSA) dismissed the performance-enhancing claims made for these drinks: there is no evidence that they delay fatigue or enhance performance. Moreover, caffeine is not recommended for children and adolescents – studies have not yet demonstrated that it is safe or effective before or during exercise. It may have unpredictable side-effects, such as trembling, rapid heartbeat, dizziness, and headaches (*see* the section on caffeine in Chapter 4, page 87). The bottom line is that young athletes should steer away from caffeine-containing energy drinks as the side-effects may outweigh the potential benefits of caffeine for performance.

The day before

On the day before competition, the focus should be on topping up glycogen stores and ensuring that they are properly hydrated. In practice, this means avoiding strenuous exercise or training that may deplete their muscle fuel stores, although light exercise may be appropriate; eating carbohydrate-rich foods at each mealtime, with a nutritious snack in between, and drinking plenty of water. Below is a checklist to help them prepare for the next day.

Top tips for the day before competition
- Eat little and often – encourage them to eat several small meals throughout the day to maximise glycogen storage.
- Avoid fatty foods – fat-rich foods and fried foods, such as burgers, pies, nuggets and chips, take longer to digest and may overburden their digestive system, making them feel sluggish the next day.
- Don't try any new foods – make sure they play it safe by sticking to familiar and plain foods; they cannot risk an upset stomach. If travelling or eating out, steer them away from anything spicy or salty, or any meat or fish that may be undercooked.
- Hydrate – they should keep a water bottle handy so they remember to drink regularly throughout the day. This is especially important if they are travelling to the competition venue on this day, as it's easy to forget to drink. Their urine should be pale in colour (*see* the 'pee chart' presented in Figure 2.1) – if not, then they need to step up their fluid intake.
- Beware of the gas – it may be wise to avoid gas-producing foods (or combinations of foods) such as beans, lentils, cruciferous vegetables (broccoli, Brussels sprouts

and cauliflower), bran cereals and spicy foods the night before the competition. They may make them feel uncomfortable the next day.

- Don't over-indulge – too much food can play havoc with the digestive system and keep them awake at night. They should keep supper light, otherwise they risk feeling heavy and sluggish the next day.
- Get organised – don't rely on finding the right foods at food outlets en route nor at the venue. It's best that the young athletes take their own supplies for the journey as well for race day. They should also take extra water in case of delays.

Competition day

What they eat and drink on the day of the competition can make a big difference to young athletes' performance. If they have followed the nutrition rules presented above over the last few days, they should arrive at the competition fully fuelled and well hydrated. But don't let them think it no longer matters what they eat, and that it's OK to indulge in sugary snacks. Too much sugar could play havoc with their blood glucose levels and result in flagging energy, fatigue and poor performance. For best performance, it's crucial that they continue paying attention to their food and drink intake before and during competition.

Eating before competing will help top up muscle glycogen stores and keep blood glucose levels steady during the competition. It is also important to replace fluids lost overnight.

Encourage them to have either a pre-competition meal or snack, depending on the start time. For early-morning starts, a normal-sized meal may not be feasible. Instead, they should eat a carbohydrate-rich meal the night before and then a healthy carbo-hydrate-rich snack (*see* the box entitled 'Pre-competition snacks') about an hour before competing. This strategy will ensure they have enough fuel for the event.

If competitors feel nervous, encourage them to consume at least a small amount of food or a liquid meal (*see* the box entitled 'How to cope with pre-competition nerves'), otherwise they risk low blood glucose levels while competing, light-headedness and a poor performance.

Top tips for competition day
- They should eat 2–4 hours before competing – eating a carbohydrate-rich pre-event meal means that they will start exercise fully fuelled.
- Avoid fry-ups – steer them away from anything fried or high in fat, such as sausages, bacon, croissants and pastries. These foods take longer to digest (especially for competitors feeling nervous) and may sit heavy in their stomach, making them feel uncomfortable during the competition. Try porridge, toast, cereal, milk, fruit or yoghurt.

HOW TO COPE WITH PRE-COMPETITION NERVES

It's very common for young athletes to get pre-competition 'nerves', which can dampen their appetite and make them feel nauseous. If they find it difficult to eat food during this time, try:

- liquid meals such as flavoured milk, sports drinks, milkshakes, yoghurt drinks and fruit smoothies;
- smooth, semi-liquid foods such as puréed fruit, yoghurt, porridge, custard and rice pudding;
- bland foods such as porridge or rice cakes.

- Drink plenty – encourage them to have a drink upon waking. If possible, they should aim to drink 400–600 ml of water or diluted fruit juice (equal amounts of juice and water) during the two-hour period before the competition. This will allow sufficient time for the fluid to get absorbed and any excess to be excreted. As a hydration check, the urine should be pale in colour before competing (*see* Figure 2.1).

- Plan an eating strategy – if they will be competing later in the day, or in several heats or matches, help them plan when to eat. Schedule meals and snacks around competition times; aim to leave two to four hours after a meal before competing, or about an hour after consuming a snack. Discourage skipping meals or constant grazing on sugary snacks otherwise their blood glucose may dip just before competing.

Q: WILL SWEETS AND CONFECTIONERY HELP GIVE YOUNG ATHLETES EXTRA ENERGY WHEN COMPETING?

A: It's very common to see young athletes grazing on sweets, jellies, glucose tablets and confectionery before competitions and during tournaments. Some are even encouraged to do so by well-meaning coaches and parents. However, the belief that these foods provide quick energy and benefit performance is unfounded. Eating too much sugar can cause big fluctuations in blood sugar levels and can, ironically, result in fatigue. Sugary foods and drinks produce a rapid rise in blood sugar levels, which in turn triggers the release of insulin to remove sugar from the bloodstream. Too much insulin can result in low blood sugar levels, light-headedness, nausea and early fatigue during exercise. Rather than giving them extra energy, sugar may sap their energy! If they need an energy boost while competing, opt for high-carbohydrate foods with a lower glycaemic index, such as bananas, dried fruit and cereal bars, that won't play havoc with their blood sugar levels. Grazing on sugary foods and drinks also increases the risk of tooth decay and acid erosion (dissolving) of the tooth enamel.

PRE-COMPETITION BREAKFASTS
- Porridge with dried fruit and honey
- Cereal with milk and yoghurt
- Scrambled egg on toast
- Toast with honey, plus yoghurt or a milky drink

PRE-COMPETITION SNACKS
- Dried fruit, e.g. raisins, apricots
- Cereal bar
- Smoothie made with fruit and yoghurt
- Yoghurt
- Milkshake or milky drink
- Banana

Q: HOW CAN I MAKE SURE PLAYERS DRINK ENOUGH DURING LONG MATCHES?

A: Playing for longer than an hour can result in significant losses of fluid, which increases the risk of dehydration, early fatigue and a drop in performance. Avoid this by encouraging the players to start the match well hydrated (the 'pee test' is a good way for them to self-monitor their hydration, *see* Figure 2.1) and to drink during breaks. Help them plan a drinking strategy – drink little and often during and immediately after the warm-up and during breaks in play. They should keep a drinks bottle handy, close to the pitch or playing area, somewhere within easy reach. If possible, they should take regular sips (or gulps), ideally every 15–20 minutes, depending on the sport, but without interrupting play! They should plan to start drinking as early as possible in the game and not wait until they feel thirsty before they start drinking.

Tournaments and multiple events

Many sporting competitions involve multiple games or a series of heats and finals on the same day or over consecutive days. To compete at their best, young athletes have to be prepared for different scenarios, and should have a flexible eating and drinking strategy, as the number of heats or games to be played may not be known, as this often depends on the outcome of individual heats and games. To further complicate matters, the exact start time of the event may change; or matches could go on for a shorter or longer duration than expected.

Turkey stir-fry with noodles

Makes 4 servings

300 g noodles
1 tablespoon olive oil
400 g turkey breast, cut into strips
2 salad onions, trimmed, washed and
diagonally sliced
2 garlic cloves, chopped
1 large carrot, cut into matchstick strips
200 g spring cabbage, sliced into 2 cm pieces
Juice of 1 lime

1   Bring a large pan of water to the boil, add
    the noodles and cook according to the
    packet instructions. Drain and transfer to
    a bowl.
2   Rub a little oil around a wok or large
    non-stick frying pan, then place over a
    high heat. Add the turkey strips and stir-fry
    for 8–10 minutes until golden and
    thoroughly cooked. Transfer to a plate,
    cover and keep warm.
3   Reheat the pan. When hot, add the
    remaining ingredients, except the turkey,
    noodles and lime juice. Stir-fry for 2
    minutes until the cabbage has wilted.
    Return the turkey and noodles to the pan
    and stir in the lime juice.
4   Serve immediately.

Nutrition (per serving)
433 kcal
33 g protein
8.3 g fat (<1 g saturates)
60 g carbohydrate

Chicken salad pitta with yoghurt dressing

Makes 4 servings

4 skinless chicken breast fillets
300 g low-fat yoghurt
Salt and freshly ground pepper
1 teaspoon ground cumin
Juice of ½ lemon
2 garlic cloves, crushed
2 teaspoons clear honey
4 wholemeal pitta breads
75–100 g mixed salad leaves
100 g cucumber, chopped
½ red pepper, deseeded and sliced
Handful fresh coriander leaves

1   Cut each chicken breast into 4–5 slices.
    Measure 100 g of the yoghurt into a bowl.
    Season and add a little of the cumin. Add
    the chicken, coat well, cover and marinate
    for 1–2 hours if possible.
2   Heat a grill or griddle pan to
    medium–high and grill the chicken,
    turning halfway through, for about 8
    minutes, or until cooked through and
    golden. Leave to cool a little. Meanwhile,
    mix the remaining yoghurt and cumin, the
    lemon juice, garlic and honey, and season.
3   Halve and split the pittas, and fill with
    some of the salad leaves and cucumber.
    Divide the chicken between the pittas,
    spoon the dressing over, and garnish with
    the pepper and coriander. Serve with any
    spare salad on the side.

Nutrition (per serving)
389 kcal
43 g protein
3.9 g fat (1.1 g saturates)
49 g carbohydrate

Tomato and tuna pasta

Makes 4 servings

225 g can tuna steak in olive oil
1 onion, finely sliced
1 garlic clove, chopped
1 red or yellow pepper, chopped
2 x 400 g cans chopped tomatoes
2 tablespoons tomato purée
300 g penne pasta
2 tablespoons basil leaves, roughly torn
20 g Parmesan

1 Drain the oil from the tuna into a medium pan and put the tuna to one side.
2 Heat 1 tablespoon of the oil and fry the onion on a low heat for about 10 minutes, until softened. Add the garlic and cook for 1 minute. Add the peppers and tinned tomatoes, and stir everything together. Simmer over a medium heat for 15 minutes to reduce the sauce.
3 Meanwhile, bring a large pan of lightly salted water to the boil and cook the pasta according to the packet instructions. Drain and toss with the sauce. Garnish with basil and Parmesan shavings, if using, to serve.

Nutrition (per serving)
458 kcal
26 g protein
13 g fat (2.7 g saturates)
63 g carbohydrate

Chilli con carne

Makes 4 servings

1 tablespoon olive oil
2 onions, chopped
1 garlic clove, chopped
2 carrots, peeled and grated
2 sticks celery, chopped
450 g lean minced beef
½ teaspoon chilli powder
A little dried oregano
3 tablespoons tomato purée
410 g can red kidney beans
400 ml water

1 Heat the olive oil in a large saucepan, add the onions, garlic, carrots, celery and mince, and cook for about 5 minutes until the mince has browned and the onion softened. Add the chilli powder and oregano, and cook for another 1–2 minutes.
2 Add the tomato purée, beans and water, cover and cook over a low heat for about 1 hour. Serve the chilli with cooked rice.

Nutrition (per serving)
250 kcal
19 g protein
11 g fat (3.2 g saturates)
19 g carbohydrate

Chicken bake

Makes 4 servings

1 tablespoon olive oil
2 onions, roughly chopped
1 garlic clove, crushed
2 x 400 g cans chopped tomatoes
125 g button mushrooms
3 courgettes, sliced
A handful of fresh basil
8 chicken thighs

1 Preheat oven to 200°C/fan 180°C/gas mark 6. Heat the oil in a frying pan, add the onions and cook for 2 minutes, then add the garlic and 50 ml water, and simmer for 3–4 minutes until soft.
2 Place the onion mixture into a roasting tin with the tomatoes, mushrooms and courgettes, then scatter with the basil leaves. Add the chicken thighs and turn to coat in the tomato mixture. Bake for 40–45 minutes, until the chicken is thoroughly cooked through and the juices run clear. Serve with cooked rice or boiled new potatoes.

Nutrition (per serving)
237 kcal
28 g protein
12 g fat (2.8 g saturates)
6.0 g carbohydrate

Rice with chicken and green beans

Makes 4 servings

400 g can cream of chicken soup
150 g long-grain rice, rinsed
500 g skinless chicken breast fillets, cut into bite-sized pieces
250 g frozen green beans
1 tablespoon chopped fresh chives

1 Tip the soup into a wide, deep frying pan, fill the can with water and rinse out into the pan. Stir in the rice and chicken, and bring to the boil. Simmer, uncovered, for 15–17 minutes, stirring occasionally, until the sauce has reduced and the rice and chicken are just cooked.
2 Meanwhile, cook the frozen beans according to the packet instructions. Fold through the chicken and rice with the chives, and season with salt and freshly ground black pepper.

Nutrition (per serving)
377 kcal
41 g protein
8.0 g fat (1.7 g saturates)
37 g carbohydrate

Tuna pasta salad

Makes 4 servings

300 g pasta shapes
4 ripe tomatoes, roughly chopped
175 g frozen peas
1 tablespoon olive oil
2 handfuls of baby spinach leaves
1 teaspoon balsamic vinegar
210 g can tuna in water, drained
Small handful basil leaves, roughly torn

1 Cook the pasta in a large pan of boiling water, according to the packet instructions.
2 Meanwhile in a small pan combine the tomatoes, peas and olive oil. Heat gently for 5 minutes.
3 Stir the baby spinach leaves and balsamic vinegar into the tomato mixture.
4 Drain the pasta and tip back into the pan, then add the vegetables, tuna and basil. Stir to combine and serve.

Nutrition (per serving)
373 kcal
23 g protein
5.0 g fat (<1 g saturates)
64 g carbohydrate

Chicken with chickpeas and tomatoes

Makes 4 servings

1 tablespoon olive oil
1 onion, chopped
2 carrots, thickly sliced
2 chicken breast fillets, cut into strips (about 300 g)
400 g can chopped tomatoes
300 ml hot chicken stock
410 g can chickpeas, drained and rinsed
Handful of fresh coriander, chopped

1 Heat the olive oil in a large, heavy-based pan, and add the onion and carrots. Cover the pan and sweat the vegetables over a low heat for 10 minutes. Remove the vegetables from the pan and set them to one side. Increase the heat slightly, add the chicken strips and cook for a few minutes until golden brown.
2 Add the vegetables back to the pan, then add the tomatoes and the stock. Stir in the chickpeas, season and bring to a simmer for 20 minutes, covered, until the chicken is cooked through. Stir in the coriander, and serve with baked potatoes or crusty bread.

Nutrition (per serving)
237 kcal
29 g protein
7.4 g fat (1.3 g saturates)
15 g carbohydrate

Pasta and prawns

Makes 4 servings

350 g dried tagliatelle
3 tablespoons olive oil
3 garlic cloves, thinly sliced
350 g raw shelled tiger prawns
Zest and juice of ½ lemon
2 tablespoons tomato purée
4 tablespoons freshly chopped parsley
2 tablespoons freshly grated Parmesan

1 Cook tagliatelle in a large pan of boiling water according to the packet instructions.
2 Meanwhile, heat half the oil in a large frying pan or wok. Fry the garlic slices for 1–2 minutes, add the prawns and cook, stirring, for 2–3 minutes until they turn pink.
3 Drain the cooked pasta and add remaining olive oil, lemon zest and juice, tomato purée, parsley and prawns. Season and toss to mix. Serve immediately, sprinkled with freshly grated Parmesan.

Nutrition (per serving)
476 kcal
29 g protein
12 g fat (2.5 g saturates)
68 g carbohydrate

Quick tuna and vegetable pasta

Makes 4 servings

1 tablespoon olive oil
1 onion, sliced
300 g pasta
300 g broccoli, chopped
210 g can tuna, drained

1 Heat the olive oil in a pan. Add the onion and cook over a medium heat for 8–10 minutes until golden and soft.
2 Meanwhile, cook the pasta in a large pan of boiling water according to the packet instructions. Add the chopped broccoli to the pasta for the last 5 minutes of cooking. Drain, then tip back into the pan.
3 Add the tuna to the pasta pan with the onions and toss everything together before serving immediately.

Nutrition (per serving)
353 kcal
22 g protein
5.0 g fat (<1 g saturates)
58 g carbohydrate

Chicken and vegetable stir-fry

Makes 4 servings

1 large onion
2 large carrots
150 g baby corn
150 g mangetout
4 skinless boneless chicken breast fillets
2 tablespoons vegetable oil
1 teaspoon curry powder
120 ml chicken stock or water
2 tablespoons tomato ketchup

1 Peel, halve and thinly slice the onion. Peel and cut the carrots in half lengthways then cut into thin slices. Halve the baby corn and mangetout.
2 Cut the chicken breasts into thin strips.
3 Heat a wok or frying pan over a high heat and add the oil. Add the chicken and curry powder and stir-fry for 2–3 minutes, until the chicken is cooked through.
4 Add the onion and carrot and stir-fry for 2 minutes more. Then add the corn and mangetout and stir-fry for a further 2 minutes.
5 Add the stock and tomato ketchup and simmer for 1–2 minutes. Serve at once with cooked rice or noodles.

Nutrition (per serving)
286 kcal
40 g protein
10 g fat (2.0 g saturates)
9.4 g carbohydrate

Lancashire hotpot

Makes 4 servings

1 tablespoon olive oil
800 g lean lamb neck fillet, cut into 5 cm (2 in) pieces
1 onion, finely diced
2 carrots, finely diced
4 celery sticks, finely diced
2 leeks, thinly sliced
2 tablespoons plain flour
Freshly ground black pepper
1 tablespoon Worcestershire sauce
800 g potatoes unpeeled

1 Heat the olive oil in a large, flameproof casserole dish. Add the lamb and cook until it is brown all over. Then transfer it to a plate.
2 Reduce the heat under your casserole dish. Add the vegetables and sauté them for 10 minutes, stirring frequently.
3 Remove the casserole from the heat, add the meat, sprinkle in the flour and mix it up thoroughly. Pour in enough hot water to cover the meat and vegetables, stir well and return to the heat.
4 Preheat the oven to 180°C/fan 160°C/gas mark 4.
5 Bring your casserole to the boil, stirring often as the gravy thickens. Season and add the Worcestershire sauce. Then remove it from the heat.
6 Thinly slice the potatoes, either by hand or with a mandolin. Layer them carefully to completely cover the meat and vegetables.
7 Place the hotpot in the oven and cook for 2 hours. The potatoes should be golden on top and the gravy bubbling up nicely around the sides.

Nutrition (per serving)
487 kcal
30 g protein
21 g fat (8.5 g saturates)
48 g carbohydrate

Chicken balti

Makes 4 servings

75 g red lentils
1 tablespoon of olive oil
2 carrots
1 mango, peeled, stoned and cubed
2 tomatoes, chopped
½ teaspoon of chilli powder
1 teaspoon of ground coriander
450 g chicken breast, boned, skinned and cubed
2 tablespoons of fresh coriander, chopped

1 Place the lentils in a saucepan and add enough water to barely cover them. Bring to the boil and then simmer for about 10 minutes, until they are soft but not mushy. Drain well and set aside.
2 Heat the oil in a large non-stick frying pan. Add the carrots and cook over a medium heat for 4–5 minutes.
3 Add the mango, tomatoes, chilli powder, ground coriander and chicken. Cook for 8–10 minutes, stirring occasionally.
4 Add the cooked lentils and cook for a further 2 minutes, or until the chicken is cooked through.
5 Garnish with fresh coriander before serving with plain basmati rice or naan bread.

Nutrition (per serving)
294 kcal
39 g protein
6.8 g fat (1.6 g saturates)
21 g carbohydrate

Fish pie

Makes 4 servings

450 g boned white fish
Milk
500 g potatoes
400 g sweet potatoes
25 g butter or margarine
225 g sweetcorn
125 g frozen peas
1 tablespoon parsley, chopped

For the cheese sauce:
25 g butter or margarine
25 g plain flour
600 ml semi-skimmed milk
125 g Cheddar cheese
A little salt, freshly ground black pepper
½ teaspoon Dijon mustard

1 Preheat the oven to 200°C/fan 180°C/gas mark 6.
2 Poach the fish in just enough milk to cover, for about 5 minutes. Drain and then roughly flake the fish.
3 Peel the potatoes and sweet potatoes and cut into large chunks. Boil until tender, drain, then mash with the butter or margarine and, if necessary, a little milk until smooth.
4 Meanwhile cook the sweetcorn (if frozen) and peas in a saucepan for about 3–4 minutes, then drain and place in a deep dish along with the fish.
5 Make the cheese sauce by melting the butter or margarine in a saucepan. Stir in the flour then gradually add the milk, whisking continuously over a low heat until the sauce has thickened. Stir in most of the cheese, salt, pepper and mustard.
6 Pour the sauce over the fish and vegetable mixture, and top with the mashed potato. Scatter over the remaining cheese. Bake for 20 minutes or until golden brown.

Nutrition (per serving)
664 kcal
38 g protein
27 g fat (15 g saturates)
73 g carbohydrate

VEGETARIAN MAIN MEALS

Pizza

Makes 1 pizza

For the pizza base:
225 g strong white flour
½ sachet easy-blend yeast
½ teaspoon salt
175 ml warm water
1 tablespoon olive oil

For the tomato sauce:
1 tablespoon olive oil
1 small onion, finely chopped
1 garlic clove, crushed
1 tin (400 g) chopped tomatoes
1 tablespoon tomato purée
1 teaspoon dried basil
½ teaspoon sugar
Pinch of salt and freshly ground black pepper
125 g mozzarella, sliced or grated Cheddar cheese

Suggested toppings: sliced tomatoes, halved cherry tomatoes, sliced red or yellow peppers, sliced mushrooms, sweetcorn, sliced onion, olives, sliced courgette, baby spinach leaves, spring onion

1 If making the dough by hand, mix the flour, yeast and salt in a large bowl. Make a well in the centre and add the oil and half the water. Stir with a wooden spoon, gradually adding more liquid until you have a pliable dough. Turn the dough out on to a floured surface and knead for about 5 minutes until you have a smooth and elastic dough. Place the dough in a clean, lightly oiled bowl, cover with a tea towel and leave in a warm place for about 1 hour or until doubled in size.

2 If you are using a bread machine, place the ingredients in the tin and follow the instructions supplied with the machine.

3 Turn out the dough; knead briefly before rolling out on a surface to the desired shape. Transfer to an oiled pizza pan or baking tray and finish shaping by hand. The dough should be approx. 5 mm thick. Let the dough rise for 30 minutes.

4 Meanwhile, make the tomato sauce. Heat the oil and sauté the onion and garlic for 5 minutes. Add the chopped tomatoes, tomato purée, basil, sugar, salt and pepper. Continue to simmer for 5–10 minutes or until the sauce has thickened a little. Spread the sauce on the pizza base. Scatter over the cheese and any additional toppings from the list above.

5 Bake at 200°C/fan 180°C/gas mark 6 for 15–20 minutes until the cheese is bubbling and golden brown.

Nutrition (per ¼ pizza)
341 kcal
14 g protein
13 g fat (5.0 g saturates)
46 g carbohydrate

FOR A QUICK MEAL, TRY ANY OF THE FOLLOWING ALTERNATIVE PIZZA BASES

- Ready-made pizza base
- An English muffin, toasted and split horizontally
- Focaccia bread, halved horizontally and toasted
- Ciabatta loaf, halved horizontally and toasted
- Wholemeal or white pitta bread, split horizontally and lightly toasted
- French bread, sliced in half horizontally and toasted

Macaroni cheese

Makes 4 servings

300 g macaroni
125 g frozen peas
25 g cornflour
300 ml milk (full-fat or semi-skimmed)
½ teaspoon Dijon mustard
85 g mature Cheddar, grated
Freshly ground black pepper

1   Preheat the oven to 200°C/fan 180°C/gas mark 6.
2   Cook the macaroni in boiling water according to the packet instructions, adding the frozen peas during the last 3 minutes of cooking time. Drain.
3   Blend the cornflour with a little of the milk in a jug. Gradually add the remainder of the milk.
4   Heat the milk and cornflour mixture in a pan, stirring continuously until the sauce just reaches the boil and has thickened.
5   Remove from the heat, stir in the mustard, half the cheese and freshly ground pepper to taste.
6   Stir in the macaroni and peas. Spoon into an ovenproof dish, scatter over the remaining cheese and bake for 15–20 minutes until the top is bubbling and golden.

Nutrition (per serving)
426 kcal
19 g protein
10 g fat (5.7 g saturates)
69 g carbohydrate

Ratatouille with butternut squash

Makes 4 servings

2 onions, cut into wedges
500 g courgettes, sliced
2 peppers (1 red, 1 yellow), cut into wide strips
1 small butternut squash (about 300 g), peeled, deseeded and cut into wedges
250 g tomatoes, quartered
2–3 garlic cloves, chopped
Few sprigs fresh thyme, roughly chopped
4 tablespoons olive oil
Freshly ground black pepper
Grated Cheddar cheese

1   Preheat the oven to 200°C/fan 180°C/gas mark 6.
2   Place the vegetables, tomatoes, garlic and thyme in a large, deep roasting tin. Drizzle over the olive oil and turn gently so that they are evenly coated with the oil. Roast in the oven for about 40 minutes or until the vegetables are beginning to soften and turn golden brown. Stir occasionally as they cook.
3   When the vegetables are ready, remove from the oven and season with freshly ground black pepper. Scatter over a little grated cheese. Serve with baked potatoes.

Nutrition (per serving)
159 kcal
3.5 g protein
12 g fat (1.8 g saturates)
10 g carbohydrate

Pasta, broccoli and cheese bake

Makes 4 servings

300 g pasta shapes
375 g broccoli
2 level tablespoons cornflour
600 ml semi-skimmed milk
½ teaspoon Dijon mustard
Freshly ground black pepper
85 g mature Cheddar cheese, grated

1 Preheat the oven to 180°C/fan 160°C/gas mark 4. Cook the pasta according to the packet instructions.
2 Cut the broccoli into small florets and boil until tender (about 5 minutes). Drain.
3 Blend the cornflour with a little of the milk in a jug. Gradually add the remainder of the milk, stirring to ensure a smooth sauce. Pour into a saucepan and heat, stirring constantly until the sauce just reaches the boil and has thickened.
4 Remove from the heat, stir in the mustard and freshly ground black pepper to taste.
5 Stir in the drained pasta and broccoli. Pour into a large ovenproof dish and scatter over the cheese. Place in the oven and bake for 20–25 minutes, until golden brown and bubbling.

Nutrition (per serving)
495 kcal
24 g protein
15 g fat (7.0 g saturates)
71 g carbohydrate

Pasta with chickpeas and spinach

Makes 4 servings

500 g fresh pasta shapes
235 g bag baby spinach
410 g can chickpeas, drained and rinsed
350 g jar tomato pasta sauce
Freshly ground black pepper
125 g cheese, grated

1 Bring a large pan of water to the boil. Add the pasta and cook according to the packet instructions. Remove from the heat and drain thoroughly. Stir in the spinach and allow to wilt.
2 Place the chickpeas in a medium pan with the tomato sauce. Gently bring to the boil over a low heat. Turn off the heat.
3 Tip the pasta into a serving dish and pour the hot pasta sauce and chickpea mixture over the top, then toss together and season with black pepper. Top each serving with grated cheese.

Nutrition (per serving)
572 kcal
28 g protein
14 g fat (5.1 g saturates)
88 g carbohydrate

Vegetarian stir-fry

Makes 4 servings

2 tablespoons light soy sauce
2 tablespoons wine vinegar
1 tablespoon sugar
1 garlic clove, crushed
350 g tofu, cut into chunks
250 g Thai fragrant rice
1 tablespoon oil
1 onion, sliced
1 red and 1 yellow pepper, deseeded and sliced
200 g broccoli, cut into florets
1 heaped teaspoon cornflour
4 tablespoons cold water
1–2 teaspoons toasted sesame seeds

1 Mix the soy sauce, vinegar, sugar and garlic, and then add the tofu and coat well. Cover and marinate for 1–2 hours if possible.
2 When ready to cook, drain the tofu, reserving the marinade. Put the rice to cook, according to packet instructions.
3 Heat a wok with half the oil over a high heat. Add the tofu (you might need to do this in batches). Stir-fry for 1–2 minutes until golden then remove to a warm plate. Add the remaining oil to the pan, then the onions, peppers and broccoli. Stir-fry for 3 minutes or until just tender.
4 Stir the cornflour and water into the reserved marinade and add to the pan, along with the tofu. Cook briefly until thickened. Add a little hot water if needed to give a rich sauce. Serve with the rice, scattered with sesame seeds.

Nutrition (per serving)
404 kcal
15 g protein
9.0 g fat (1.2 g saturates)
70 g carbohydrate

Three-bean pasta

Makes 4 servings

2 tablespoons oil
1 onion, finely chopped
1 celery stick, finely chopped
1 parsnip, chopped
1 garlic clove, crushed
1 bay leaf
400 g can mixed beans, drained
400 g can chopped tomatoes
1 tablespoon tomato purée
2 tablespoons roughly chopped herbs, such as basil, thyme, rosemary
450 ml vegetable stock
300 g small pasta shapes
25 g Parmesan, freshly grated, to serve

1 Heat the oil in a pan and add the onion, celery, parsnip and garlic. Add a splash of water and cover. Cook over a low to medium heat for 5–10 minutes until the vegetables are soft and translucent.
2 Add the bay leaf, beans, chopped tomatoes, tomato purée, herbs and stock. Season, cover and bring to the boil. Simmer for 15 minutes.
3 Add the pasta to the pan and stir. Put the lid back on and bring to a simmer. Cook for 10 minutes.
4 Remove the bay leaf and stir half the Parmesan into the pan. Spoon into bowls and sprinkle with the remaining cheese.

Nutrition (per serving)
455 kcal
18 g protein
9.7 g fat (2.4 g saturates)
79 g carbohydrate

Pasta and tomato salad

Makes 4 servings

300 g dried pasta shapes
2 tablespoons olive oil
4 sun-dried tomatoes in oil, drained
4–5 spring onions
225 g cherry tomatoes
8–12 basil leaves
8–12 black olives
125 g mature Cheddar cheese, cut into cubes

1　Cook the pasta in a large pan of boiling water until al dente, according to the packet instructions. Drain the pasta, refresh under cold running water, then drain again and transfer to a large bowl. Stir in the olive oil to prevent the pasta from sticking.
2　Slice the sun-dried tomatoes. Trim and finely shred the spring onions. Halve the cherry tomatoes. Tear the basil leaves into pieces. Add to the pasta along with the olives and toss to mix.
3　Toss with the cubes of cheese and accompany with a leafy green salad

Nutrition (per serving)
378 kcal
9.9 g protein
13 g fat (1.9 g saturates)
59 g carbohydrate

Roast tomato pasta

Makes 4 servings

300 g dried pasta
500 g cherry tomatoes
2 tablespoons olive oil
Salt and freshly ground black pepper
60 g pine nuts
A large handful of basil leaves, torn
Freshly grated Parmesan cheese

1　Preheat the oven to 240°C/fan 220°C/gas mark 9.
2　Bring a large pan of water to the boil and cook the pasta according to the packet instructions. Drain the pasta well.
3　Meanwhile, cut the tomatoes in half and arrange them in a large roasting tin, cut side up. Drizzle them with olive oil. Season with salt and black pepper. Roast in the oven for 15 minutes until the tomatoes are softened and lightly caramelised. Meanwhile, put the pine nuts on to a separate roasting tray and roast for 5–7 minutes until lightly golden.
4　Mix the pasta with the tomatoes, basil and pine nuts, then stir in a little extra oil if the pasta needs it. Serve sprinkled with a generous amount of Parmesan.

Nutrition (per serving)
478 kcal
16 g protein
21 g fat (3.8 g saturates)
61 g carbohydrate

Pasta with mushrooms

Makes 4 servings

350 g pasta shapes
1 tablespoon olive oil
1 onion, sliced
200 g button mushrooms
3 tablespoons crème fraîche
2 tablespoons freshly chopped flat-leafed
parsley

1   Cook the pasta in a large pan of boiling
    water, according to the packet
    instructions.
2   Meanwhile, heat the olive oil in a pan.
    Add the sliced onions and fry gently for
    3 minutes until starting to soften. Add the
    button mushrooms and fry for 5–6
    minutes. Drain the pasta, return to the
    pan and add the onions and mushrooms.
3   Stir in the crème fraîche and parsley. Toss
    everything together, season to taste and
    heat through to serve.

Nutrition (per serving)
392 kcal
12 g protein
11 g fat (4.8 g saturates)
67 g carbohydrate

Pasta with butternut squash

Makes 4 servings

1 butternut squash, halved, peeled and
roughly chopped
2 tablespoons olive oil
Zest of 1 lemon
Salt and freshly ground black pepper
350 g pasta shapes
75 g Cheddar cheese, grated
Fresh basil leaves, torn

1   Preheat the oven to 200°C/fan 180°C/gas
    mark 6.
2   Place the butternut squash in a roasting
    pan, drizzle with olive oil and add the
    lemon zest. Sprinkle with a little salt and
    freshly ground black pepper. Cook in the
    oven for about 20 minutes, until soft and
    the edges just begin to colour.
3   In a large pan of boiling water, cook the
    pasta according to the packet instructions,
    drain and tip back into the pan with a little
    of the cooking water. Toss with the roasted
    squash, then stir through the cheese and
    more black pepper if needed. Scatter with
    fresh basil to serve.

Nutrition (per serving)
458 kcal
16 g protein
14 g fat (5.1 g saturates)
73 g carbohydrate

Pesto pasta with vegetables

Makes 4 servings

300 g pasta shapes
50 g pine nuts
1 tablespoon olive oil
1 crushed garlic clove
250 g sliced mushrooms
2 sliced courgettes
250 g cherry tomatoes
3 tablespoons pesto
25 g Parmesan

1   Cook the pasta according to the packet instructions.
2   Gently toast the pine nuts in a frying pan for a few minutes. Remove. Add olive oil to the pan, then the garlic, mushrooms and courgettes. Add a splash of water to the pan, then cover and cook for 4–5 minutes. Uncover and add cherry tomatoes, then cook for a further 1–2 minutes.
3   Drain the pasta and return to the pan. Add the vegetables and pine nuts, the pesto and Parmesan to the drained pasta. Toss well to combine, and serve immediately.

Nutrition (per serving)
527 kcal
20 g protein
25 g fat (5.0 g saturates)
61 g carbohydrate

Vegetable pasta bake

Makes 4 servings

225 g pasta shapes
2 large carrots, thinly sliced
175 g broccoli, cut into small florets
125 g tinned sweetcorn
1 tablespoon olive oil
60 g Cheddar cheese, grated
1 tablespoon sunflower seeds, toasted
60 g fresh breadcrumbs

For the cheese sauce:
1 level tablespoon cornflour
300 ml semi-skimmed milk
½ teaspoon Dijon mustard
60 g mature Cheddar cheese, grated
Freshly ground black pepper

1   Preheat oven to 200°C/fan 180°C/gas mark 6.
2   Cook the pasta shapes according to the packet instructions. Drain and transfer to an ovenproof dish.
3   Place the carrots in a pan of boiling water and cook for 3 minutes. Add the broccoli and cook until just tender. Drain well.
4   Make the cheese sauce. Blend the cornflour with a little of the milk in a jug. Gradually add the remainder of the milk, stirring to ensure a smooth sauce. Pour into a saucepan and heat, stirring constantly until the sauce just reaches the boil and has thickened.
5   Remove from the heat, stir in the mustard, cheese and freshly ground black pepper to taste. Stir the cooked vegetables, sweetcorn and cheese sauce into the pasta and season.
6   Mix the oil, cheese and sunflower seeds into the breadcrumbs, then scatter over the vegetables. Cook in the oven for 20 minutes, until the topping is golden.

Nutrition (per serving)
537 kcal
21 g protein
19 g fat (8.2 g saturates)
76 g carbohydrate

Bean and vegetable stew

Makes 4 servings

1 tablespoon olive oil
225 g mushrooms
2 carrots, sliced
1 large potato, cubed
225 g green beans, chopped
1 teaspoon dried thyme
2 garlic cloves, crushed
700 ml vegetable stock
Seasoning
225 g frozen broad beans
410 g can borlotti beans (or any other variety of beans)

1 Heat the oil in a large pan, add the mushrooms, carrots, potato and green beans, and gently fry for 3–4 minutes.
2 Add the thyme, garlic and vegetable stock. Bring to the boil, then simmer uncovered for 20 minutes until the vegetables are tender.
3 Stir in all the beans and then cook for a further 10 minutes. Serve with baked potatoes.

Nutrition (per serving)
224 kcal
12 g protein
6.8 g fat (1.0 g saturates)
31 g carbohydrate

Thai vegetable curry

Makes 4 servings

400 ml can reduced-fat coconut milk
2 tablespoons Thai green curry paste
2 carrots, sliced
300 g broccoli, divided into small florets
150 g sugar snap peas, trimmed
150 g baby sweetcorn, cut in half
100 g unsalted cashew nuts

1 Pour the coconut milk into a wide pan, then stir in the green curry paste and bring to a simmer.
2 Add the carrots and simmer gently for 10 minutes.
3 Add the broccoli florets, sugar snap peas and sliced baby sweetcorn, and simmer gently for a further 5 minutes.
4 Stir in the cashew nuts, and serve with boiled rice or rice noodles.

Nutrition (per serving)
243 kcal
11 g protein
15 g fat (2.8 g saturates)
17 g carbohydrate

Vegetable chilli

Makes 4 servings

2 tablespoons oil
1 onion, sliced
2 red peppers, deseeded and cut into chunks
1 tablespoon mild chilli powder
1 large carrot, peeled and cut into chunks
2 medium potatoes, peeled and cut into chunks
400 g can chopped tomatoes
200 ml hot vegetable stock
410 g can red kidney beans in chilli sauce
50 g green beans, trimmed and halved

1   Heat the oil in a large pan. Add the onion and cook on a medium heat for 5 minutes until softened, then add the peppers and cook for 2 minutes. Add the chilli powder and stir for 1 minute. Stir in the carrot and potatoes, then add the tomatoes and stock and simmer for 15–20 minutes.
2   Add the red kidney beans and simmer for a further 5 minutes. Finally, add the green beans and simmer for 5–10 minutes or until all the vegetables are tender. Serve with basmati rice.

Nutrition (per serving)
249 kcal
9.0 g protein
6.8 g fat (1.0 g saturates)
40 g carbohydrate

Vegetable risotto

Makes 4 servings

15 g butter
1 tablespoon olive oil
2 red peppers, sliced
300 g risotto rice
1 clove garlic, crushed and chopped
750 ml hot vegetable stock
200 g runner beans
125 g spinach
50 g Parmesan shavings

1   Melt butter and oil in a pan, add the peppers, rice and garlic. Mix well. Add a ladleful of hot stock and stir well, simmer and repeat until all stock is added and the rice is just cooked.
2   Slice beans and add for the final 3 minutes of cooking. Stir in the spinach and serve topped with Parmesan.

Nutrition (per serving)
420 kcal
12 g protein
11 g fat (4.9 g saturates)
72 g carbohydrate

SOUP

Vegetable soup

Makes 4 servings

2 tablespoons olive oil
1 onion, chopped
1 garlic clove, crushed
1 litre vegetable stock
750 g vegetables, e.g. sliced carrots, diced
butternut squash, green beans, frozen peas,
broccoli florets, cauliflower florets
Salt and freshly ground black pepper
1 tablespoon fresh herbs, e.g. chives, parsley,
basil, thyme

1 Heat the olive oil in a large pan. Add the
   onion and garlic and cook for about
   5 minutes. Add the stock and the prepared
   vegetables, bring to the boil and then
   simmer for about 20 minutes or until the
   vegetables are soft.
2 Turn off the heat. Season and stir in the
   herbs.
3 For a smooth soup, liquidise in a blender
   or food processor, or using a hand
   blender. For a chunky, thick soup, liquidise
   half the soup and return to the pan.

Nutrition (per serving)
115 kcal
1.3 g protein
6.1 g fat (1.0 g saturates)
15 g carbohydrate

Butternut squash soup

Makes 4 servings

2 tablespoons olive oil
1 onion, chopped
1 medium (about 450 g) butternut squash,
peeled and chopped
1 large carrot, sliced
1 medium potato, peeled and chopped
900 ml vegetable stock
1 teaspoon (5 ml) grated fresh ginger (or
½ teaspoon ground ginger)
Freshly ground black pepper

1 Heat the oil and sauté the onion for about
   5 minutes, until transparent.
2 Add the butternut squash, carrot and
   potato, and cook for a further
   2–3 minutes.
3 Add the stock and grated ginger and bring
   to the boil. Turn down the heat and
   simmer for 20 minutes or until the
   vegetables are tender.
4 Remove from the heat. Liquidise the soup
   using a hand blender or food processor.
5 Season with black pepper.

Nutrition (per serving)
143 kcal
2.5 g protein
5.9 g fat (<1 g saturates)
21 g carbohydrate

Carrot and coriander soup

Makes 4 servings

1 tablespoon (15 ml) extra virgin olive oil
1 onion, finely sliced
1 garlic clove, crushed
500 g carrots, sliced
700 ml vegetable stock
1 bay leaf
Salt and freshly ground black pepper
A handful of fresh coriander, roughly chopped

1 Heat the olive oil in a heavy-based saucepan over a moderate heat. Add the onion and sauté gently for about 5 minutes until it is translucent.
2 Add the garlic and cook for a further 1–2 minutes. Add the carrots, stock and bay leaf to the pan, stir, then bring to the boil. Simmer for 15 minutes or until the vegetables are tender.
3 Allow the soup to cool slightly for a couple of minutes. Remove and discard the bay leaf. Liquidise the soup using a hand blender or conventional blender. Season to taste, then stir in the fresh coriander.

Nutrition (per serving)
93 kcal
<1 g protein
5.9 g fat (1 g saturates)
9.9 g carbohydrate

Pea soup

Makes 4 servings

Knob of butter
1 tablespoon olive oil
1 small onion, finely chopped
Salt and freshly ground pepper
600 ml vegetable stock
400 g fresh or frozen peas
A handful of mint leaves, roughly chopped
4 tablespoons low-fat yoghurt, to serve

1 Melt the butter with the oil in a large saucepan over a medium heat. Add the onion, season, cover and cook very gently for 15 minutes or until completely soft.
2 Add the stock and bring to a gentle simmer, then add the peas and simmer for 10 minutes until they are soft. Remove from the heat, add the chopped mint, and purée.
3 Serve hot or chilled, garnished with a swirl of yoghurt, a sprig of mint and lots of black pepper, accompanied by crusty wholemeal bread.

Nutrition (per serving)
141 kcal
7.6 g protein
7.1 g fat (2.8 g saturates)
12 g carbohydrate

Lentil soup

Makes 4 servings

2 tablespoons olive oil
1 large onion, chopped
1–2 garlic cloves, crushed
225 g red lentils
1 litre vegetable stock
Juice of 1 lemon
Salt and freshly ground black pepper

1   Heat the olive oil in a heavy-based saucepan over a moderate heat. Add the onion and garlic and cook for about 5 minutes until translucent.
2   Add the lentils and vegetable stock, and bring to the boil. Reduce the heat and simmer for 20 minutes. Add the lemon juice, bring back to the boil and simmer for a further 10 minutes until the lentils are soft.
3   Season to taste, ladle into bowls.

Nutrition (per serving)
228 kcal
13 g protein
6.2 g fat (<1 g saturates)
32 g carbohydrate

Tomato soup

Makes 4 servings

2 tablespoons olive oil
1 onion, chopped
1 large carrot, grated
1 red pepper, chopped
1 large potato, peeled and cubed
2 garlic cloves, crushed
1 tin (400 g) chopped tomatoes
750 ml boiling water or hot vegetable stock
1 teaspoon (5 ml) sugar
Freshly ground black pepper

1   Heat the oil and sauté the onion for 2–3 minutes in a large saucepan. Add the carrot, red pepper, potato and garlic, and cook for a further 5 minutes.
2   Add the tomatoes, water and sugar. Simmer for about 20 minutes or until the vegetables are soft.
3   Liquidise the soup using a hand blender or food processor, and season with the black pepper.

Nutrition (per serving)
125 kcal
2.4 g protein
5.9 fat (<1 g saturates)
16 g carbohydrate

DESSERTS

Apple crumble

Makes 4 servings

700 g cooking apples
2 tablespoons caster sugar
2 tablespoons water
2 teaspoons ground cinnamon
100 g plain flour
50 g light brown sugar
50 g porridge oats
50 g butter or margarine

1 Preheat the oven to 190°C/fan 170°C/gas mark 5.
2 Peel, core and thinly slice the apples, and place in a 1-litre pudding basin. Toss with the sugar. Pour over 2 tablespoons boiling water.
3 Place the cinnamon, flour, brown sugar and oats in a mixing bowl. Add the butter or margarine and rub in to the mixture until it resembles breadcrumbs.
4 Sprinkle the topping over the apples and bake for 40–45 minutes until golden brown. Serve with a spoonful of home-made custard.

Nutrition (per portion)
271 kcal
7.4 g protein
9.2 g fat (4.6 g saturates)
42 g carbohydrate

Apple pancakes

Makes 4 servings

100 g self-raising flour
2 eggs, beaten
150 ml milk
3 tablespoons caster sugar
Small amount of oil
25 g butter or margarine
2 eating apples, thinly sliced

1 Put the flour in a mixing bowl, make a well in the centre, add the eggs and a little milk, and mix to a smooth paste. Slowly add the rest of the milk and beat to a smooth batter. Stir in 1 tablespoon of the caster sugar.
2 Lightly oil a frying pan and heat. Drop a large tablespoonful of mixture on to the hot pan, cook for 2–3 minutes until golden brown underneath and almost set on top, turn over and cook other side until golden. Keep warm while making remaining pancakes.
3 Melt the butter or margarine in a small frying pan and fry the apple slices until golden. Add the remaining sugar and stir until dissolved. Serve with the pancakes.

Nutrition (per portion)
378 kcal
4.5 g protein
12 g fat (6.6 g saturates)
68 g carbohydrate

Baked bananas with apricots

Makes 4 servings

4 bananas
125 g ready-to-eat dried apricots
1 tablespoon honey
4 tablespoon toasted flaked almonds

1 Preheat the oven to 190°C/fan 170°C/gas mark 4. Cut four rectangles of foil, 25 x 30 cm each.
2 Peel the bananas. Split in half lengthways, not quite cutting all the way through. Place each one on a piece of foil.
3 Put the apricots into a food processor. Add 4 tablespoons of water and the honey, and process for a few seconds to make a smooth purée.
4 Spoon the purée over the bananas and fold over the foil, twisting the ends to make sealed parcels. Arrange on a baking tray and bake for 10 minutes.
5 Carefully open the foil parcels and scatter over the almonds.
6 Serve with yoghurt or ice cream.

Nutrition (per portion)
235 kcal
4.6 g protein
6.1 g fat (<1 g saturates)
43 g carbohydrate

Oat, banana and yoghurt pots

Makes 4 servings

6 tablespoons porridge oats
2 tablespoons sugar
2 bananas
400 ml natural yoghurt

1 Sprinkle the oats on a baking tray with the sugar. Grill gently for 3–4 minutes, turning frequently until golden and crisp.
2 Mash the bananas and mix with the yoghurt. Layer into four tumblers with the toasted oats.

Nutrition (per portion)
203 kcal
7.3 g protein
2.5 g fat (<1 g saturates)
40 g carbohydrate

Plum clafoutis

Makes 4 servings

500 g plums
20 g butter
25 g plain flour
25 g caster sugar
3 eggs
350 ml semi-skimmed milk

1 Heat the oven to 180°C/fan 160°C/gas mark 4.
2 Halve the plums and remove the stones. Butter a shallow baking dish and add the plums.
3 In a blender, mix the flour, caster sugar, eggs and milk until smooth and creamy.
4 Pour over the plums and bake in the oven for 30–35 minutes.
5 Leave to cool a little and then dust lightly with sugar.

Nutrition (per portion)
235 kcal
10 g protein
11 g fat (5.0 g saturates)
27 g carbohydrate

Rice pudding

Makes 4 servings

50 g pudding rice
600 ml milk (full-fat or semi-skimmed)
40 g sugar
Grated nutmeg

1 Preheat the oven to 150°C/fan 130°C/gas mark 2.
2 Put the rice, milk and sugar in a 1.8-litre pie dish. Stir the mixture, then sprinkle with grated nutmeg.
3 Bake for 1½ hours, or until the milk has been absorbed and there is a light-brown skin on top of the pudding. Serve with spicy fruit compote (*see* recipe, page XX) or tinned apricots.

Nutrition (per portion)
154 kcal
5.9 g protein
2.7 fat (1.6 g saturates)
28 g carbohydrate

Baked apples

Makes 4 servings

4 Bramley cooking apples
60 g sultanas
6–8 ready-to-eat dried apricots, chopped
1 tablespoon clear honey
2 tablespoons pecans, chopped

1 Preheat the oven to 190°C/fan 170°C/gas mark 5.
2 Remove the core from the apples. Using a sharp knife, lightly score the skin around the middle, just enough to pierce the skin.
3 In a small bowl, combine the dried fruit, honey and pecans. Fill the cavities of the apples, then place them in a baking dish. They should fit snugly side by side. Add 2 tablespoons of water, cover loosely with foil then bake for 45–60 minutes.
4 Check a few times during cooking, adding a little extra water if the dish becomes dry.
5 Serve warm with natural yoghurt.

Nutrition (per portion)
284 kcal
4.3 g protein
9.3 g fat (<1 g saturates)
49 g carbohydrate

Spicy fruit compote

Makes 4 servings

1 tablespoon clear honey
1 teaspoon ground cinnamon
Juice of 1 lemon
500 g dried fruit, e.g. apricots, apples, pears, prunes, figs and cranberries, roughly chopped

1 Put the honey, cinnamon, lemon juice and 600 ml boiling water in a large pan. Bring to the boil and simmer for 5 minutes. Add the dried fruit and then simmer for a further 5 minutes. Remove from the heat and leave to steep until ready to serve.
2 Serve with yoghurt or vanilla ice cream.

Nutrition (per portion)
226 kcal
5.0 g protein
<1 g fat (<1 g saturates)
53 g carbohydrate

BAKING

Honey flapjacks

Makes 12 slices

200 g butter or margarine
200 g sugar
200 g honey
400 g porridge oats
50 g sultanas or glacé cherries

1 Preheat the oven to 180°C/fan 160°C/gas mark 4. Grease a 20 x 30 cm cake tin.
2 Put the butter, sugar and honey in a saucepan and heat, stirring occasionally, until the butter has melted and the sugar has dissolved. Add the oats and sultanas or cherries, and mix well.
3 Transfer the oat mixture to the prepared cake tin and spread to about 2 cm thick. Smooth the surface with the back of a spoon.
4 Bake in the oven for 15–20 minutes, until lightly golden around the edges but still slightly soft in the middle.
5 Let cool in the tin, then turn out and cut into squares.

Nutrition (per slice)
383 kcal
4.3 g protein
17 g fat (2.8 g saturates)
57 g carbohydrate

Banana and walnut loaf

Makes 10 slices

2 medium bananas
125 g butter
175 g dark brown sugar
2 eggs
1 teaspoon vanilla essence
1 teaspoon ground cinnamon
250 g plain flour
1 teaspoon baking powder
3 tablespoons milk
125 g walnuts

1 Preheat the oven to 180°C/fan 160°C/gas mark 4. Grease a 1 kg loaf tin or use 12 large muffin cases.
2 Mash the bananas. Cream the butter and sugar until smooth and then beat in the mashed bananas. Add the eggs, vanilla and cinnamon, and mix well.
3 Add the flour, baking powder and milk, and mix until smooth. Fold in the walnuts.
4 Spoon the mixture into the tin and bake for about 50 minutes, until the loaf is crusty on the top and a skewer inserted into the middle comes out clean. Cool in the tin and then turn out on to a cooling rack. For muffins, cook for 20–25 minutes.

Nutrition (per slice)
370 kcal
6.0 g protein
21 g fat (7.7 g saturates)
43 g carbohydrate

Blueberry muffins

Makes 18 muffins

375 g flour
1 tablespoon baking powder
150 g caster sugar
2 large eggs
90 g melted butter
284 ml pot of buttermilk
200 g blueberries

1   Preheat the oven to 200°C/fan 180°C/gas mark 6 and line two 12-hole muffin trays with paper cases.
2   Sift the flour and baking powder into a large bowl and stir in the sugar.
3   In another bowl, whisk together 2 large eggs, melted butter and a pot of buttermilk. Fold this mixture into the flour and stir the blueberries through. Spoon into paper cases and bake for 20–25 minutes until cooked and golden.

Nutrition (per muffin)
152 kcal
2.8 g protein
5.1 g fat (2.9 g saturates)
25 g carbohydrate

Fruit buns

Makes 12 buns

500 g strong white bread flour
1 teaspoon salt
2 teaspoons mixed spice
100 g caster sugar
7 g sachet easy-blend dried yeast
100 g dried mixed fruit
50 g butter
250 ml milk, plus 3 tablespoons milk
1 large egg, beaten

1   In a large bowl, sift together the flour, salt, spice and 50 g of the sugar, stir in the yeast and fruit. In a small pan, melt the butter, then add the milk and heat until tepid – it should just feel warm to the touch.
2   Make a well in the dry ingredients, stir in the milk, then the egg, and mix to form a soft dough. Tip the dough out on to a floured work surface and knead for 5–8 minutes until smooth and elastic.
3   Divide into 12 equal pieces and shape each into a ball. Place a little way apart on an oiled baking sheet, use a knife to cut a cross in top of each. Cover with oiled clear film and leave to prove in a warm place for about 1½ hours until doubled in size.
4   Preheat the oven to 190°C/fan 170°C/gas mark 5. Bake for 20–25 minutes or until golden brown.
5   When the buns are nearly ready, heat the remaining sugar and milk with 3 tablespoons water in a small pan, stirring until the sugar dissolves. Boil for 1 minute. Remove the buns from the oven and brush with the glaze. Leave to cool on a wire rack. Serve warm, spread with butter.

Nutrition (per bun)
246 kcal
6.4 g protein
4.9 g fat (2.6 g saturates)
47 g carbohydrate

Raspberry muffins

Makes 12 muffins

4 tablespoons sunflower oil
75 ml milk
1 large egg
150 g self-raising flour
100 g caster sugar
175 g fresh or frozen raspberries
4 tablespoons icing sugar, sifted
2 teaspoons lemon juice

1 Preheat the oven to 200°C/fan 180°C/gas mark 6. Line a six-hole deep muffin tray with paper cases.
2 Mix the oil, milk and egg together. Sift the flour and sugar into a bowl. Add the liquid and half the raspberries to the flour and briefly mix until just coming together. Spoon into the muffin cases and scatter over the remaining raspberries. Bake for 25–30 minutes.
3 Cool the muffins on a wire rack. Sift the icing sugar into a bowl, stir in lemon juice to make a runny icing. Drizzle the icing over the muffins and leave to set. Pack the muffins into an airtight container. They will keep for 2–3 days.

Nutrition (per muffin)
145 kcal
2.0 g protein
4.5 g fat (<1 g saturates)
26 g carbohydrate

Almond and apricot cake

Makes 12 slices

150 g margarine
150 g sugar
2 eggs
100 g ground almonds
175 g self-raising flour
300 ml plain low-fat yoghurt
100 g ready-to-eat apricots

1 Preheat the oven to 180°C/fan 160°C/gas mark 4. Line a 20 cm round cake tin with baking parchment.
2 Beat the margarine and sugar until pale and creamy.
3 Add the eggs, almonds, flour and yoghurt, and combine well.
4 Roughly chop the apricots and then fold in to the mixture.
5 Spoon in to the prepared tin and bake in the oven for 30–40 minutes or until a skewer inserted in to the centre comes out clean. Leave to cook in the tin for 10 minutes, remove from the tin and cool on a wire rack.

Nutrition (per slice)
284 kcal
5.9 g protein
17 g fat (3.0 g saturates)
30 g carbohydrate

Date slice

Makes 12 slices

350 g pitted dates
200 ml water
A piece of lemon rind
150 g butter or margarine
225 g wholemeal flour
125 g rolled oats
85 g brown sugar

1 Preheat the oven to 200°C/fan 180°C/gas mark 6. Oil a rectangular tin, 28 x 18 cm.
2 Place the dates, water and lemon rind in a small saucepan, bring to the boil and simmer for 8–10 minutes, until very soft. Discard the peel.
3 Rub the butter or margarine into the flour until the mixture resembles breadcrumbs. Stir in the oats and sugar.
4 Press half the crumble mixture into the prepared tin. Spread the dates over and then cover with the remaining crumble.
5 Bake in the preheated oven for 20–25 minutes or until lightly browned. Cut into 16 slices.

Nutrition (per slice)
255 kcal
4.2 g protein
12 g fat (6.6 g saturates)
36 g carbohydrate

Chocolate chip oat cookies

Makes 20 cookies

125 g butter or margarine
85 g brown sugar
85 g granulated or caster sugar
1 egg
½ teaspoon vanilla essence
150 g plain white flour
½ teaspoon baking powder
60 g rolled oats
100 g chocolate chips

1 Preheat the oven to 180°C/fan 160°C/gas mark 4 and oil one or two baking sheets (or use baking parchment).
2 Cream together the butter or margarine and the sugars until light and smooth.
3 Beat in the egg and vanilla.
4 Mix the flour and baking powder together, then add along with the oats to the mixture, mixing well. Stir in the chocolate chips.
5 Place spoonfuls on to the baking sheets, about 2.5 cm apart, and bake for 8–10 minutes or until lightly browned. Allow to cool for about 5 minutes before gently lifting with a spatula on to a wire rack.

Nutrition (per cookie)
146 kcal
1.8 g protein
7.2 g fat (4.2 g saturates)
20 g carbohydrate

Fruit loaf

Makes 10 slices

300 ml/½ pint milk
175 g golden caster sugar
75 g dried vine fruit
250 g dried apricots or plums, chopped, or
use more dried vine fruit
3 tablespoons golden syrup
2 tablespoons runny honey
350 g self-raising flour, sifted
1–2 tablespoons ground ginger or mixed
spice, sifted
3 tablespoons apricot jam

1 Preheat the oven to 180°C/fan 170°C/gas
   mark 4. To a large bowl, add the milk and
   sugar, then mix in the fruit. Drizzle in syrup
   and honey, and stir well. Next, add the
   flour and spice, and mix again until
   combined.
2 Spoon into a loaf tin and place in the oven
   for about 45 minutes to an hour, until
   golden brown and a skewer comes out
   clean when poked in the middle. Leave to
   cool in the tin for 10 minutes before
   turning out on to a wire rack. Melt a little
   apricot jam and brush it over the cake.
   Slice to serve.

Nutrition (per slice)
317 kcal
5.1 g protein
1.1 g fat (<1 g saturates)
76 g carbohydrate

Wholemeal bread

Makes 16 slices

500 g strong wholemeal bread flour
1 teaspoon salt
1 teaspoon fast-action dried yeast
1 teaspoon sugar
1 tablespoon olive oil
325 ml warm water

1 In a large bowl, mix together the flour,
   salt, yeast and sugar. Add the oil and
   water, and roughly mix into the flour. Stir
   together until you have a soft dough.
2 Lightly flour your hands and the work
   surface. Transfer the dough on to the work
   surface and knead well for about 10
   minutes until it feels smooth and pliable.
3 Leave the dough covered with a tea towel,
   in a draught-free place, for it to double in
   size (this should take about an hour).
4 Turn the dough out on to a floured surface
   and knead the dough firmly for several
   minutes.
5 Shape the dough and put it into an oiled
   1 kg bread tin, or place it on an oiled
   baking sheet.
6 Cover with a clean tea towel and leave the
   dough to rise for about 25 minutes in a
   warm place. Preheat the oven to 220°C/
   fan 200°C/gas mark 7.
7 Bake in a preheated oven for 35–40
   minutes. It should sound hollow if tapped
   on the base.

Nutrition (per slice)
103 kcal
4.0 g protein
1.4 g fat (<1 g saturates)
20 g carbohydrate

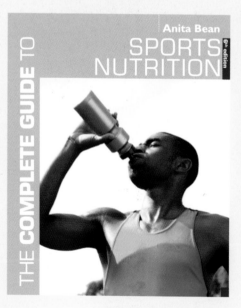

Food for Fitness
ANITA BEAN

Food for Fitness is the bible for anyone who takes their sport, health and fitness seriously. It is packed full of information on nutrition – clearly distinguishing between myth and reality – and includes ten ready-made meal plans, plus guidance on how to develop your own. It also contains over 50 recipes for snacks, meals and drinks.

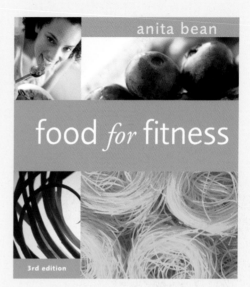

Healthy Eating for Kids
ANITA BEAN

Packed with essential up-to-date advice on healthy eating, feeding fussy eaters, dealing with an overweight child, and plenty of tips for no-hassle meals, quick snacks and lunch boxes, including brand new colour photographs of the recipes. Tested by parents and tasted by children, Anita's recipes will give you new idea and inspiration on what to feed your kids.

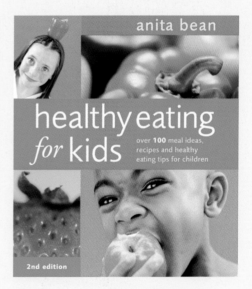